Management of Menopause
in Cancer Survivors

As perceptions of menopause have evolved, this new text examines what clinical problems can arise in treatment of patients experiencing menopause after cancer treatment. For too long, menopausal symptoms have been undertreated in cancer survivors, leading to suffering and suboptimal health outcomes. From hot flashes to night sweats to mood and sexual concerns, this book provides practical tips for approaching these symptoms in the clinic. It will be an invaluable reference for both gynaecologists and oncologists internationally.

Management of Menopause in Cancer Survivors

Edited by

Swati Jha MD, FRCOG

Subspecialist in Urogynaecology at Sheffield Teaching Hospitals and
Honorary Professor at the University of Sheffield, UK

Lidia Schapira MD

Professor of Medicine (Oncology), Stanford University School of Medicine,
Stanford, California, USA

CRC Press
Taylor & Francis Group
Boca Raton London

CRC Press is an imprint of the
Taylor & Francis Group, an **informa** business

Designed cover image: Shutterstock image id 2250879569

First edition published 2026
by CRC Press
2385 NW Executive Center Drive, Suite 320, Boca Raton FL 33431

and by CRC Press
4 Park Square, Milton Park, Abingdon, Oxon, OX14 4RN

CRC Press is an imprint of Taylor & Francis Group, LLC

© 2026 selection and editorial matter, Swati Jha and Lidia Schapira; individual chapters, the contributors

ISBN: 978-1-032-63100-4 (hbk)
ISBN: 978-1-032-62620-8 (pbk)
ISBN: 978-1-032-63102-8 (ebk)

DOI: 10.1201/9781032631028

Typeset in Garamond
by Apex CoVantage, LLC

Contents

Preface

For most of human history, menopause may have been seen as a developmental transition. In the past couple of centuries, menopause became a subject of medical interest starting in Europe, and today it is a topic of conversation in professional and informal forums across the world. Natural menopause may be viewed as a part of the life cycle and reproductive strategy that is unique to humans. Medical menopause, that is menopause deliberately induced as part of a therapeutic plan, is typically more abrupt and premature in a woman's life cycle. Medical menopause may trigger a series of physical and emotional symptoms that have a profound and negative impact on many dimensions of quality of life.

As physicians specializing in gynaecology and oncology, we have seen the gamut of physiological and psychosocial adverse effects of medical menopause. We have listened to patients and accompanied friends as they made decisions about their bodies that they knew would impact their future health and wellbeing. For patients with hormonally sensitive cancers for whom medical menopause was prescribed as treatment, managing side-effects may be especially challenging.

With growing numbers of cancer survivors, the need to offer state-of-the-art menopause care and symptom relief has become a focus for cancer multidisciplinary teams. There are many problems and syndromes that require attention, including fertility and family building considerations, pelvic floor problems, genitourinary symptoms, intimacy and sexual wellbeing, bone health, sleep disturbances and mood changes. These problems may be exacerbated for marginalized groups, including sexually diverse populations and those with a prior history of stigma and discrimination.

In this book we look at a range of issues relating to cancer care and the consequences of menopause either caused by the cancer treatment or impacting its treatment. Starting with physiology, epidemiology, cultural variations and navigating genetic cancer risk, the book then addresses both pharmacological and non-pharmacological options for symptom treatment of menopause. Fertility issues, a consequence of early cancer diagnosis, are addressed in considerable detail with a range of options and their success discussed. There is a separate chapter that addresses the needs of breast cancer survivors, because this is the most common cancer in women, and often treatment itself exacerbates menopausal symptoms. The book also delves into options for sexual health and intimacy as well as management of pelvic floor problems, both of which can be impacted by accelerated menopause as a result of cancer treatment.

We are most grateful for the contributions to this book of colleagues with expertise in treating menopausal symptoms. Each chapter examines a particular population and problem, and offers advice that is informed by evidence and clinical experience. We hope that you will find this useful in your practice and, above all, that it will help individuals struggling to regain their wellbeing after having been treated for cancer.

The motivation to write this book stems from the editors' professional experience of managing these problems on a day-to-day basis and, for one of the editors (SJ), their own personal experience of dealing with cancer.

—**Swati Jha and Lidia Schapira**

Contributors

Ruth Athey
Urogynaecology
Sheffield Teaching Hospitals NHS Foundation
  Trust
Sheffield, UK

Daniel S. Childs
Department of Oncology
Mayo Clinic
Rochester, MN, USA

Darya Dahi
Emory University
Atlanta, GA, USA

Kirsten Das
Eunice Kennedy Shriver National Institute
  of Child Health and Human Development
Bethesda, MD, USA

Rhianna Davies
Gynaecology
Queen Charlotte's and Chelsea Hospitals
London, UK

Don S. Dizon
Pelvic Malignancies Program, The Cancer
  Center
Brown University Health and Legorreta Cancer
  Institute and Brown University
Providence, RI, USA

Claudine Domoney
Gynaecology
Chelsea and Westminster Hospital
London, UK

Christine A. Duffy
Adult Survivorship Services
The Cancer Center at Brown University Health
Providence, RI, USA

Mridula A. George
Rutgers Cancer Institute
The State University of New Jersey
New Brunswick, NJ, USA

Ana Ferrigno Guajardo
Yale Cancer Center
Yale School of Medicine
New Haven, CT, USA

Tim Hillard
Gynaecology
University Hospitals Dorset
Poole, Dorset, UK

Kang Woo Kim
Department of Medicine, Alpert Medical School
Brown University
Providence, RI, USA

Charles L. Loprinzi
Department of Oncology
Mayo Clinic
Rochester, MN, USA

Maryam B. Lustberg
Internal Medicine (Medical Oncology), Breast
  Medical Oncology
Center for Breast Cancer, Yale University
  School of Medicine
New Haven, CT, USA

Jacqueline C. Yano Maher
Eunice Kennedy Shriver National Institute
    of Child Health and Human
    Development
Bethesda, MD, USA

Jane Meisel
Department of Hematology and Medical
    Oncology
Department of Gynecology and
    Obstetrics
Winship Cancer Institute
Emory University School of
    Medicine
Atlanta, GA, USA

Nick Panay
Gynaecology
Queen Charlotte's and Chelsea Hospitals
London, UK

Hana R. Rosenow
Department of Medicine
Mayo Clinic
Rochester, MN, USA

Elle Sein
Institute of Reproductive and Developmental
    Biology
Imperial College
London, UK

Alexa Steckler
Alpert Medical School
Brown University
Providence, RI, USA

Elizabeth Varghese
Eunice Kennedy Shriver National Institute
    of Child Health and Human Development
Bethesda, MD, USA

Chapter 1

Physiology of Menopause

Rhianna Davies and Nick Panay

Introduction

With increasing life expectancy, a significant portion of a woman's life will be during and after the menopause transition. Symptoms affect 80% of women, with severe symptoms in one third (1). The menopause transition can have a considerable impact on women's mood, relationships, ability to work and quality of life (2). For those also navigating life with a new cancer diagnosis, or experiencing troublesome symptoms of treatment or its sequelae, there may be additional considerations (3, 4). Furthermore, the use of systemic hormone replacement therapy (HRT) may be contra-indicated.

Natural menopause is a retrospective diagnosis following 12 months of amenorrhoea in the absence of pathological explanation; the average age in the UK is 51 years old (5). It is derived from the Greek *menos*, meaning month, and *pausis*, meaning an ending. The age of natural menopause is understood to be influenced by many factors including body mass index, socio-economic background, parity, ethnicity and genetics (6). Additionally, factors such as surgery or chemoradiotherapy can accelerate the age of menopause (7). Natural menopause is predated by a period, often years, of irregular periods and the onset of symptoms as ovarian reserve dwindles. In comparison, surgically or chemically induced menopause may subvert this gradual transition. The change in hormone levels that occurs during the menopausal transition, especially oestradiol, can cause physical menopause symptoms including vasomotor symptoms such as hot flushes and night sweats, dry skin and hair and musculoskeletal aches. Many women also report psychological symptoms such as mood changes and anxiety. Interestingly, there are cultural and geographical differences in which symptoms tend to predominate.

Physiology of the Natural Menopausal Transition

Women are born with their lifetime supply of ovarian follicles. From menarche to menopause a tightly regulated cyclical pattern of hormonal change occurs to induce monthly ovulation. The hypothalamo-pituitary-gonadal axis is governed primarily by the hormones gonadotropin releasing hormone (GnRH), follicle stimulating hormone (FSH), luteinising hormone (LH), oestradiol

DOI: 10.1201/9781032631028-1

and progesterone (5). FSH and LH, produced by the anterior pituitary under the pulsatile control of hypothalamic GnRH, orchestrate oestradiol and progesterone production from the ovaries. FSH stimulates oestradiol production from the ovarian follicles (5). Oocyte numbers decline with advancing age, and at a critical level cessation of ovarian response induces the changes associated with menopause (1, 8). FSH, and later LH, levels increase to maintain normal circulating oestradiol levels. Declining follicles and thus the ability to produce oestradiol in response to FSH result in progressively anovulatory cycles leading to irregular menses. FSH levels fluctuate dramatically during the menopausal transition, often day to day, limiting diagnostic value (9). Ultimately oestradiol production is insufficient to stimulate endometrial proliferation and amenorrhoea ensues (5).

Other notable hormones derived from the ovary include the peptide inhibin B which exerts negative feedback on gonadotropins, anti-mullerian hormone (AMH), a peptide growth factor produced by the ovarian granulosa cells in the early follicular development stage, and androgens. AMH levels, relatively stable throughout the menstrual cycle, fall as ovarian function declines. Its clinical predictive value for fertility potential or onset of menopause is currently limited (4). Both the ovaries and adrenal glands produce androgenic precursors to testosterone including androstenedione and dehydroepiandrosterone (DHEA). Testosterone can be hydroxylated to dihydroprogesterone or aromatised to oestradiol. The mean serum levels of testosterone, androstenedione and DHEA of a woman in her mid-40s are about 50% of those of a woman in her 20s (10, 11). Low serum testosterone has been proposed to induce low sexual desire, often associated with menopause; however, there is limited evidence for a correlation between androgen levels and sexual desire in women (10, 11). Indeed, menopausal status does not appear to affect levels of androgens in women aged 45–54 years old, and both the adrenal glands and postmenopausal ovary continue to produce androgens (11).

As the menopausal transition progresses oestradiol, inhibin B and AMH levels decrease, whilst gonadotropin levels increase (1, 8). In the absence of ovulation, progesterone levels remain at the follicular phase low levels. There is inadequate oestrogenic stimulation of the endometrium, and menses cease. Testosterone levels do not change as significantly during the early menopausal transition, and thus the relatively elevated androgen:oestrogen ratio results in the signs of androgen excess seen in some women during this period (8). The symptoms and ramifications of menopause are manifold and can be broadly separated into acute symptoms and long-term health concerns resulting from low oestrogen.

Menstrual Disturbance

Preceding the final menstrual period, perimenopause is characterised by cycles of increasingly variable length (12). Increasingly frequent anovulatory cycles allow the build-up of endometrium and can result in heavy withdrawal bleeds when they do occur (1).

Vasomotor Symptoms

Vasomotor symptom is a term that encompasses hot flushes, transient periods of intense heat in the upper half of the body with associated sweating, and night sweats. Hot flushes can be associated with palpitations and anxiety, and can be followed by chills (13). The severity and frequency of vasomotor symptoms vary widely amongst women; they are the most commonly reported symptom of menopause amongst Caucasian women (2). Whilst often starting prior to amenorrhoea, the prevalence of hot flushes is highest in the first year after the final menstrual period (10). Vasomotor symptoms affect 75% of women, with 29% classing them as severe. The median duration of vasomotor symptoms is 7 years (10). The pathology of vasomotor symptoms is not fully understood, but it is considered likely due to a narrowing of the thermoneutral zone at the level of the hypothalamus (13). Various neurotransmitters such as kisspeptin, serotonin and noradrenaline have been proposed to contribute to the causation of low oestrogen and vasomotor symptoms (5, 10, 14). However not all women with low oestrogen levels will develop vasomotor symptoms; thus, it is likely that other factors play a causative role. Ethnic variation may be accounted for by genetics, socio-cultural and dietary differences (5, 15). Vasomotor symptoms can disturb sleep, resulting in poor energy levels and lower mood, as well as impaired quality of life (16).

Cognitive, Psychological and Sleep Symptoms

Cognitive function appears to decline during the menopausal transition, often described by women as brain fog (5). Women specifically report reduced focus, impaired memory and reduced speed of thought (17). Objective testing has found that premenopausal women outperform postmenopausal women on formal neuropsychological testing (18). Oestrogen has established effects in the brain on metabolism, neurotransmission and increased cerebral blood flow (19).

Many women report anxiety, irritability, low mood, mood swings, tiredness and feeling overwhelmed during the menopausal transition. Whilst similar mood changes are noted at other times of hormonal alternation such as premenstrually and postnatally, the exact mechanisms are unclear. Studies report a greater risk of depression in peri- and postmenopausal women compared with premenopausal women (1). Additionally, 40% of women report sleep disturbance during the menopausal transition (20). The Study of Women's Health Across the Nation (SWAN) found association between low oestrogen levels, depression and anxiety symptoms, vasomotor symptoms and disturbed sleep (21). The exact mechanisms of menopause-related insomnia remain unclear, but it cannot be accounted for by night sweats alone (20). A holistic approach to the patient is therefore vital because psychological symptoms at this life stage may be multi-factorial including, or exacerbated by, life events.

Urogenital Syndrome of Menopause

Urogenital syndrome of menopause describes the resultant atrophy, change in integrity and decreased secretory function of the lower urinary and genital tract in response to low sex steroids. Patients report vaginal and vulval dryness, itching and soreness, as well as urinary urgency, frequency, incontinence and propensity for urinary tract infections (22, 23). The urinary and genital tract have a common embryological origin and both are densely populated with oestrogen receptors (24). Oestrogen acts upon these receptors to induce vasodilation of blood vessels and proliferation of the vaginal epithelium. Alongside secretions from the Bartholin's and endocervical glands, fluid transudate from dilated blood vessels forms the vaginal secretions and thus lubrication (23). The vaginal epithelium produces glycogen, which is converted to glucose to nourish the vaginal bacteria flora. Lactobacilli metabolise glucose to lactic and acetic acids, hence the low vaginal pH (25). Vaginal acidity provides an immune function, reducing the rates of vaginal and urinary tract infection (23).

Low oestrogen causes the vaginal epithelium to become thin, pale and prone to petechial haemorrhage. Lower vaginal lactic acid production increases vaginal pH thereby increasing the risk of pathogenic alterations to the vaginal flora (26). Reduced vaginal and cervical secretions can cause reduced lubrication and thus painful sex. About 40–54% of postmenopausal women reported symptoms of genitourinary syndrome of menopause (27). However, the symptoms are potentially underreported due to embarrassment (28). Clinician-reported examination findings have been found to be associated with symptom severity and quality of life impairment (29).

A vulva and vagina with atrophic epithelium and reduced lubrication can lead to dyspareunia (25). Indeed, the tissue may fissure following penetration (25). Interest in sex declines in women with age, which can cause relationship difficulties (30). The loss of libido described during the menopausal transition is not fully explained by vulvo-vaginal atrophy, nor concurrent life stressors, and may also have a hormonal component (30). The British Menopause Society supports a trial of transdermal testosterone in well-oestrogenised (via conventional HRT) postmenopausal women with hypoactive sexual desire disorder (HSDD), provided other causes such as relationship issues, psychosexual problems and medication-related HSDD have been ruled out (31). Testosterone treatment in postmenopausal women is currently off-license in most parts of the world, although a 1% testosterone cream is licensed in Australia.

Atrophy of the urethra and bladder can lead to urinary frequency and incontinence (32, 33). Evidence suggests a lack of oestrogen decreases the sensory threshold for bladder distention, impairs urethral closure pressure and impairs connective tissue integrity of the urethral sphincter leading to stress urinary incontinence (24, 34). Topical oestrogen usually relieves local symptoms, avoids hepatic metabolism and is associated with little to no systemic absorption (25). Evidence suggests vulvo-vaginal application of topical oestrogen decreases vaginal pH, increases lactobacilli, improves tissue integrity in the vagina, urethra and urethral sphincter, and reduces urinary frequency, urgency, stress incontinence and recurrent UTI (35).

Long-Term Sequelae of Menopause

Cardiovascular disease, resulting in coronary heart disease (CHD) and stroke, is the leading cause worldwide of death in men and women (10). Oestrogen is known to be protective against cardiovascular disease; premenopausal women have a lower risk of CHD than age-matched males. However, women catch up with male rates of CHD after the age of menopause, mainly as a consequence of declining oestrogen levels (10).

The healthy skeleton continuously remodels via osteoclasts (bone resorption) and osteoblasts (bone formation); this is crucial for adequate bone mineral density (36). Oestrogen is pivotal for this via various mechanisms including lowering the sensitivity of bone to the parathyroid hormone and stimulating the production of calcitonin to reduce bone resorption, reducing renal calcium excretion, and increasing gastrointestinal calcium resorption (36). Oestrogen deficiency thus impairs the normal bone renewal cycle. Osteoclast-driven resorption increases whilst osteoblast-driven bone formation decreases, leading to bone loss (36).

The incidence of dementia is higher in women than men (37). This incidence cannot be fully explained by the average longer life expectancy of women. It is currently unclear whether the cognitive impairment reported by women during the menopausal transition persists into older age. Multiple trials have investigated whether HRT reduces the rates of dementia with conflicting results, perhaps due to confounding by other underlying risk factors (38).

Menopausal Symptoms during or after Cancer Treatment

The management of cancer can lead to either transient or permanent cessation of ovarian function. Surgical removal of the ovaries in cases of ovarian cancer, or risk-reduction for groups such as BRCA mutation carriers at increased risk of ovarian cancer, results in both abrupt and permanent cessation of ovarian function. Both systemic chemotherapy and either pelvic radiotherapy or total body irradiation can result in ovarian failure (7). Importantly, and unpredictably, in the case of chemotherapy- or radiotherapy-induced ovarian failure, spontaneous ovulation may resume many years later (39). There is no current way to predict for whom menopause may be permanent, but it is more likely with increasing age at which chemotherapy was administered (40, 41). A meta-analysis of 45 studies of female cancer survivors, diagnosed from childhood to 40 years old, found the average age of menopause to be 44 years old (42). The cornerstone of management for some hormone-sensitive cancers is medical hormonal blockade; this will introduce menopause symptoms for the period of time that they are used.

Menopause symptoms in cancer patients can differ significantly from those experienced during natural menopause due to the influence of cancer treatments, the abruptness of hormonal changes and the unique psychological and physical challenges faced by individuals undergoing cancer therapy. Understanding these differences is essential for providing targeted care and support strategies for women undergoing menopause in the context of cancer treatment.

Abrupt Onset and Premature Menopause

The abrupt onset of surgical or chemically induced menopause can intensify symptoms and make the adjustment to menopause more challenging. Vasomotor symptoms are reported as more severe in women who have had breast cancer treatment than those who have not (43). Greater than 90% of women who have undergone a bilateral oophorectomy will encounter vasomotor symptoms due to abrupt decrease in oestradiol (44). In contrast the natural menopause typically occurs gradually over several years, allowing women to adapt to hormonal changes more slowly. Similarly the abrupt withdrawal of oestrogen can lead to greater degrees of sexual dysfunction than the gradual withdrawal of the natural menopausal transition (25). Surgical menopause is considered to induce a more pronounced negative impact on executive function and memory than the natural menopause (45). Animal models of oophorectomy show plausibility of low oestrogen leading to altered brain metabolism, oxidative stress, dendritic growth and cerebral blood flow (46). Studies suggest surgical menopause results in greater impairment in quality of life outcomes than natural menopause (25).

Variability in Symptoms

The severity and onset of symptoms in cancer-induced menopause can vary widely depending on the type of cancer, the stage of the disease and the specific treatments administered. The cornerstone of management of oestrogen receptor positive breast cancer is the use of endocrine therapies designed to block or reduce the proliferative action of oestrogen on breast tissue. This can, however, lead to reduced circulating oestrogen accessible to other oestrogen receptors such as those in the genito-urinary system. Aromatase inhibitors in particular can cause significant symptoms of vulval atrophy (47). Furthermore, the most commonly reported side effect of adjuvant endocrine therapy is vasomotor symptoms (48). Indeed, up to 20% of women either stop or consider stopping their adjuvant endocrine therapy due to menopausal side effects (49).

Control of symptoms is thus vital to adherence to recurrence-reducing therapy. However, use of HRT may be counter-intuitive to the aim of reducing oestrogen. Tamoxifen and aromatase inhibitors both reduce exposure of breast tissue to oestrogen. Aromatase inhibitors work primarily by inhibition of peripheral androgen conversion to oestrogen by >95% (50). In contrast, tamoxifen works by selective blockage of estrogen receptors. It has a degree of positive oestrogenic action in the vagina, similar to its action in the endometrium, and thus causes fewer symptoms of vaginal dryness (47, 48).

Aggravation of Menopausal Symptoms

The intensity of menopausal symptoms may be heightened in cancer patients due to the overall physical and emotional toll of cancer treatments. Cancer patients undergoing menopausal symptoms may experience heightened emotional distress due to the dual burden of cancer diagnosis and treatment-related hormonal fluctuations. The psychological impact can be significant, affecting mental well-being and quality of life. Compared to natural menopause, the emotional burden in cancer-induced menopause is often compounded by the stress and uncertainty of cancer treatment. For women on HRT who are diagnosed with a de novo malignancy, initial advice often includes cessation of possibly causative HRT and thus re-introduction of prior menopausal symptoms (51). Furthermore, breast cancer is the most common cancer in perimenopausal women, and thus menopausal symptoms may coincide naturally with a diagnosis of breast cancer (3). All this is compounded by the possible adverse effects of chemotherapy, radiotherapy and any adjuvant treatments.

Overlap of Symptoms

Distinguishing symptoms of menopause from those specifically associated with cancer treatment is a crucial aspect in providing personalised care. Hair loss, brain fog and tiredness may be encountered both in menopause and as a direct effect of cancer treatment (52). The emotional and physical challenges associated with a cancer diagnosis create a complex interplay of factors that influence various aspects of a woman's mental health (53).

The initial phase following a cancer diagnosis may be shock and denial, leading to heightened stress, anxiety, mood disturbance and sleep disruption. The fear of the unknown or anxiety about an uncertain future may antagonise this. The physical and emotional demands of cancer treatment, coupled with the stress of the diagnosis itself, contribute to cancer-related fatigue. Poor sleep, physical discomfort relating to surgery, nausea and distress can lead to cognitive impairment, difficulty concentrating, decline in memory and difficulties with decision making. This can affect a woman's ability to perform daily tasks and contribute to a sense of frustration and helplessness. A cancer diagnosis can alter social relationships, leading to potential feelings of isolation and changes in dynamics within families and friendship groups. Disruption to a support network may further exacerbate low mood and anxiety (54).

Cancer treatment can have a profound effect on a woman's libido and sexual function. As in natural menopause, cessation of ovarian function induced by cancer treatment or surgery can result in vaginal atrophy, superficial dyspareunia and low libido. Furthermore, pelvic radiotherapy can damage the surrounding vasculature and nerves, resulting in reduced blood flow or sensation (55). Hysterectomy alters the anatomy of the pelvis and may reduce lubrication or sensation during intercourse. Many women report loss of orgasmic function following hysterectomy (56). Hysterectomy and thus loss of reproductive capacity may have a profound impact on a woman's psychological well-being, leading to a sense of loss, grief or bereavement for what might have been. It may lead to a change in personal identity, especially a loss of femininity (57). Similarly, a mastectomy may lead to a feeling of loss of attractiveness or desirability for some (58). Breast surgery may lead to loss of nipple sensation and thus decreased sexual pleasure and feelings of intimacy. Cancer treatment can lead to other physical changes such as scars, hair loss or colostomies, which may further impact body image, self-esteem and confidence (59). Emotional well-being is closely associated with sexual health in women. Cancer-related fatigue and treatment-related pain may result in loss of sexual desire. Medication such as anti-depressants to manage either menopausal symptoms or cancer-related mood changes can lead to sexual dysfunction (57). The dynamics of a relationship often change when one is ill; it may be a challenge for a partner to revert to being a lover when they have acted as a carer (57). There can be communication barriers between women and their doctors because the patient may fear reporting sexual dysfunction in the context of surviving cancer to be trivial (57). The psycho-sexual ramification of cancer treatment may be complex, involving physical, emotional and interpersonal challenges (55–59).

Management Options during Cancer Treatment

Different cancers carry different risk profiles in terms of their hormonal sensitivity status, and for many, evidence is lacking for the safety of HRT use entirely. It is generally considered that systemic HRT should be avoided in breast and ovarian cancer (60, 61), that it can be used in bowel, haematological, vulval, vaginal and squamous cell carcinoma, which are hormone receptor-negative, and that there is no consensus for malignant melanoma (53).

Furthermore, management strategies for hormone-sensitive cancers are themselves the direct cause of the hypoestrogenic state, e.g. aromatase-inhibitors. Non-hormonal prescription alternatives for vasomotor or mood symptoms are available, but caution must be taken in patients using tamoxifen (31). Some drugs can compete for metabolism via the CYP2D6 pathway, lowering the plasma concentrations of tamoxifen thereby increasing the risk of breast cancer recurrence. Vulval symptoms may be improved with physiological moisturisers for comfort or lubricants for sex (62). Pelvic floor physiotherapy, vaginal dilators and psychosexual counselling may have benefit (57). Over-the-counter magnesium, the Sleepio app and sleep hygiene advice can be helpful (63). Over-the-counter vitamin D may be important for bone support. Cognitive behavioural therapy (CBT) for menopause, mindfulness, yoga, acupuncture and meditation may have value but high-quality randomised controlled trials are needed (64, 65). Pre-operative counselling and post-operative support are crucial. Patient support groups may offer valuable comfort and sources of advice during this uncertain time (66). Lifestyle modifications such as reduced alcohol, nicotine and caffeine and increased exercise reduce vasomotor symptoms and improve quality of life (65); it must be borne in mind that advice such as increased exercise may not be realistic or appropriate for patients dealing with treatment-related fatigue.

Conclusion

The multi-faceted nature of cancer-induced menopause necessitates a comprehensive and person-alised approach. Recognising the interconnectedness of physical and emotional well-being, as well as appreciating the overlap and mutual exacerbation between menopausal symptoms, the effect of a cancer diagnosis and the impact of cancer treatment, is crucial to achieve a holist approach to care. This involves collaboration between different medical specialists, thorough patient communication and a nuanced understanding of the unique needs and challenges faced by women experiencing menopausal symptoms whilst undergoing cancer therapies.

References

1. O'Neill S, Eden J. The pathophysiology of menopausal symptoms. Obstet Gynaecol Reprod Med. 2012;22(3):63–9.
2. Hamoda H et al. The British Menopause Society & Women's Health Concern 2020 recommendations on hormone replacement therapy in menopausal women. Post Reprod Health. 2020;26(4):181–209.
3. Hickey M et al. Practical clinical guidelines for assessing and managing menopausal symptoms after breast cancer. Ann Oncol. 2008;19(10):1669–80.
4. Panay N, Fenton A. Iatrogenic menopause following gynecological malignancy: Time for action! Climacteric. 2016;19(1):1–2.
5. Santoro N et al. The menopause transition: Signs, symptoms, and management options. J Clin Endocrinol Metab. 2021;106(1):1–15.
6. Gold EB. The timing of the age at which natural menopause occurs. Obstet Gynecol Clin N Am. 2011;38(3):425–40.
7. Marino JL et al. Managing menopausal symptoms after cancer: An evidence-based approach for primary care. Med J Aust. 2018;208:127–32.
8. Hall JE. Endocrinology of the menopause. Endocrinol Metab Clin N Am. 2015;44(3):485–96.
9. Hale GE et al. The perimenopausal woman: Endocrinology and management. J Steroid Biochem Mol Biol. 2014;142:121–31.
10. Hillard T et al., eds. Management of the Menopause. 6th ed. Marlow: BMS; 2017.
11. Davis SR et al. Androgens and female sexual function and dysfunction—findings from the fourth international consultation of sexual medicine. J Sex Med. 2016;13(2):168–78.
12. Taffe JR, Dennerstein L. Menstrual patterns leading to the final menstrual period. Menopause. 2002;9(1):32–40.
13. Freedman RR. Pathophysiology and treatment of menopausal hot flashes. Semin Reprod Med. 2005;23(2):117–25.
14. Rance NE et al. Modulation of body temperature and LH secretion by hypothalamic KNDy (kisspeptin, neurokinin B and dynorphin) neurons: A novel hypothesis on the mechanism of hot flushes. Front Neuroendocrinol. 2013;34(3):211–27.
15. Martín Salinas C, Lopez-Sobaler A. Beneficios de la soja en la salud femenina [Benefits of soy in women's health]. Nutr Hosp. 2017;34:36–40.
16. Gracia CR, Freeman EW. Onset of the menopause transition: The earliest signs and symptoms. Obstet Gynecol Clin N Am. 2018;45(4):585–97.
17. Davey DA. Alzheimer's disease, dementia, mild cognitive impairment and the menopause: A "window of opportunity"? Women's Health. 2013;9(3):279–90.
18. Pike CJ et al. Protective actions of sex steroids. Front Neuroendocrinol. 2009;30:239–58.
19. Hogervorst E et al. Cognition and mental health in menopause: A review. Best Pract Res Clin Obstet Gynaecol. 2022;81:69–84.
20. Vivian-Taylor J, Hickey M. Menopause and depression: Is there a link? Maturitas. 2014;79(2):142–6.
21. Bromberger JT et al. Depressive symptoms during the menopausal transition: The Study of Women's Health Across the Nation (SWAN). J Affect Disord. 2007;103(1):267–72.
22. Wines N, Willsteed E. Menopause and the skin. Aust J Dermatol. 2001;42:149–58.
23. The North American Menopause Society Editorial Panel. The 2020 genitourinary syndrome of menopause position statement of the North American Menopause Society. Menopause. 2020;27(9):976–92.
24. Robinson D, Cardozo LD. The role of estrogens in female lower urinary tract dysfunction. Urology. 2003;62:45–51.
25. Gandhi J et al. Genitourinary syndrome of menopause: An overview of clinical manifestations, pathophysiology, etiology, evaluation, and management. Am J Obstet Gynecol. 2016;215(6):704–11.
26. Willhite LA, O'Connell MB. Urogenital atrophy: Prevention and treatment. Pharmacotherapy. 2001;21:464–80.
27. DiBonaventura M et al. The association between vulvovaginal atrophy symptoms and quality of life among postmenopausal women in the United States and Western Europe. J Women's Health. 2015;24:713–22.

28. Nappi RE et al. Diagnosis and management of symptoms associated with vulvovaginal atrophy: Expert opinion on behalf of the Italian VVA Study Group. Gynecol Endocrinol. 2016;32(8):602–6.
29. Palacios S et al. The European Vulvovaginal Epidemiological Survey (EVES): Prevalence, symptoms and impact of vulvovaginal atrophy of menopause. Climacteric. 2018;21(3):286–91.
30. Pettigrew JA, Novick AM. Hypoactive sexual desire disorder in women: Physiology, assessment, diagnosis, and treatment. J Midwifery Women's Health. 2021;66:740–74.
31. Woyka J. Prescribable Alternatives to HRT [internet], BMS, 2020. Available from: https://thebms.org.uk/wp-content/uploads/2022/12/02-BMS-TfC-Prescribable-alternatives-to-HRT-NOV2022-A.pdf.
32. Palacios S. Managing urogenital atrophy. Maturitas. 2009;63:315–18.
33. The North American Menopause Society Editorial Panel. The role of local vaginal estrogen for treatment of vaginal atrophy in postmenopausal women: 2007 position statement of the North American Menopause Society. Menopause. 2007;14:355–69.
34. Hyun HS et al. Urodynamic characterization of postmenopausal women with stress urinary incontinence: Retrospective study in incontinent pre- and post-menopausal women. J Korean Soc Menopause. 2010;16:148–52.
35. Cox P, Panay N. Vulvovaginal atrophy in women after cancer. Climacteric. 2019 Dec;22(6):565–71.
36. Ji MX, Yu Q. Primary osteoporosis in postmenopausal women. Chronic Dis Transl Med. 2015;1(1):9–13.
37. Chene G. Gender and incidence of dementia in the Framingham Heart Study from mid-adult life. Alzheimer's Demen. 2015;11:310–20.
38. Pertesi S et al. Menopause, cognition and dementia—a review. Post Reprod Health. 2019;25(4):200–6.
39. Sukumvanich P et al. Incidence and time course of bleeding after long-term amenorrhea after breast cancer treatment: A prospective study. Cancer Biol Med. 2010;116:3102–11.
40. Hunter MS et al. NICE guidance on Menopause: Cognitive behavioral therapy is an effective non-hormonal intervention for managing vasomotor symptoms. BMJ. 2015;351:6434.
41. Stefanopoulou E, Hunter MS. Does pattern recognition software using the Bahr monitor improve the sensitivity, specificity, and concordance of ambulatory skin conductance monitoring of hot flushes? Menopause. 2013;20:1133–8.
42. Overbeek A et al. Chemotherapy-related late adverse effects on ovarian function in female survivors of childhood and young adult cancer: A systematic review. Cancer Treat Rev. 2017;53:10–24.
43. Santoro NF. What a SWAN can teach us about menopause. Contemporary Ob Gyn. 2004;49(5):69–79.
44. Bachmann GA. Vasomotor flushes in menopausal women. Am J Obstet Gynecol. 1999;180(3):S312–16.
45. Rocca WA et al. Increased risk of cognitive impairment or dementia in women who underwent oophorectomy before menopause. Neurol. 2007;69(11):1074e83.
46. Bustamante-Barrientos FA et al. The impact of estrogen and estrogen-like molecules in neurogenesis and neurodegeneration: Beneficial or harmful? Front Cell Neurosci. 2021;15(52).
47. Howell A et al. ATAC Trialist's Group (2005) results of the ATAC trial after completion of 5 years' adjuvant treatment for breast cancer. Lancet. 2005;365:60–2.
48. Cella D, Fallowfield LJ. Recognition and management of treatment-related side effects for breast cancer patients receiving adjuvant endocrine therapy. Breast Cancer Res Treat. 2008;107:167–80.
49. Barron TI et al. Early discontinuation of tamoxifen: A lesson for oncologists. Cancer. 2007;109(5):832–9.
50. Kendall A et al. Caution: Vaginal estradiol appears to be contraindicated in postmenopausal women on adjuvant aromatase inhibitors. Ann Oncol. 2006;17(4):584–7.
51. Haskell SG. After the Women's Health Initiative: Postmenopausal women's experiences with discontinuing estrogen replacement therapy. J Women's Health. 2004;13(4):438–42.
52. Glaus A et al. Fatigue and menopausal symptoms in women with breast cancer undergoing hormonal cancer treatment. Ann Oncol. 2006;17(5):801–6.
53. Szabo RA et al. Managing menopausal symptoms after cancer. Climacteric. 2019;22(6):572–8.
54. Pinquart M, Duberstein PR. Associations of social networks with cancer mortality: A meta-analysis. Criti Rev Oncol/Hematol. 2010;75(2):122–37.
55. Jensen PT, Froeding LP. Pelvic radiotherapy and sexual function in women. Transl Androl Urol. 2015;4(2):186–205.

56. Lonnée-Hoffmann R, Pinas I. Effects of Hysterectomy on sexual function. Curr Sex Health Rep. 2014;6:244–51.

57. Brough P, Denman M. Introduction to Psychosexual Medicine. 3rd ed. Boca Raton: CRC Press; 2019.

58. Rojas K et al. The impact of mastectomy type on the Female Sexual Function Index (FSFI), satisfaction with appearance, and the reconstructed breast's role in intimacy. Breast Cancer Res Treat. 2017;163:273–9.

59. Ozturk O et al. Sexual dysfunction among patients having undergone colostomy and its relationship with self-esteem. J Family Med Community Health. 2015;2(1):1028.

60. de Villiers TJ et al. Revised global consensus statement on menopausal hormone therapy. Climacteric. 2016;19:313–15.

61. O'Donnell RL et al. Hormone replacement therapy after treatment for a gynaecological malignancy. Curr Opin Obstet Gynecol. 2016;28:32–41.

62. Edwards D, Panay N. Treating vulvovaginal atrophy/genitourinary syndrome of menopause: How important is vaginal lubricant and moisturizer composition? Climacteric. 2016;19(2):151–61.

63. Polasek D et al. Nutritional interventions in treating menopause-related sleep disturbances: A systematic review. Nutr Rev. 2023; 82(8):1087–1110.

64. Hunter M, Smith M. Cognitive Behaviour Therapy (CBT) for Menopausal Symptoms [internet], BMS, 2019. Available from: https://thebms.org.uk/wp-content/uploads/2022/12/01-BMS-TfC-CBT-NOV2022-A.pdf.

65. Woyka J. Non-Hormonal-Based Treatments for Menopausal Symptoms [internet], BMS, 2022. Available from: https://thebms.org.uk/publications/consensus-statements/non-hormonal-based-treatments-menopausal-symptoms/.

66. Weis J. Support groups for cancer patients. Support Care Cancer. 2003;11:763–8.

Chapter 2

Cultural Variations of Menopause

Ruth Athey and Swati Jha

Introduction

The transitional period of menopause marks a major health landmark for women. Although we often focus on the symptoms during menopause and the perimenopausal period, the biological, psychological, social and behavioural changes during this period shape women's health into later life (1). These have been discussed in detail in the first chapter.

The impact of menopause is a spectrum with differing impacts on women depending on several factors. The Fawcett Society report of 2022 (2) identified differences in access to care and treatment in ethnic minorities within the workplace. Some studies have shown that there are differences in the changes of hormone levels and physical symptoms experienced around the time of menopause for women from different racial, ethnic and cultural backgrounds (3). There are significant variations, with women's perceptions, attitudes and expectations about menopause being significantly influenced by external factors including cultural background (3). Women from ethnic minorities may lack awareness of perimenopause and menopausal symptoms.

When examining the impact of culture on menopause, historically there have been two prevailing views in research. Some researchers have taken the approach that the biological changes associated with menopause are universal and that the variable factors are women's perceptions and social experiences. Another school of thought is that different genetic, social and cultural factors interact in complex ways that are currently poorly understood, leading to different individual experiences (3). Different factors associated with culture such as diet, climate, ecology, patterns and expectations associated with childbirth or fertility may also play a role, to a greater or lesser extent (4).

When examining these differences, we must be careful when assigning or designating cultures based on ethnic background or location. Culture is not necessarily bound by geographical, ethnic or national demarcations, and when asking about cultural and ethnic background, it is important to ask about self-assigned cultural affiliations. It is also important to assess how much an individual identifies with or participates in the values of the dominant culture to which they assign themselves (3).

DOI: 10.1201/9781032631028-2

The understanding of menopause is shaped by cultural perspectives, and there is a complex interplay between ethnicity and culture as well as attitudes towards menopause. There have been multiple studies into ethnic variations of menopause, but very little published literature on the variations of an iatrogenic menopause induced by cancer treatment. This chapter will therefore rely predominantly on evidence from research into the former.

Ethnicity also impacts how people cope with cancer, and there have been wide variations identified in awareness of symptoms and barriers to help seeking amongst different ethnic groups (5). This will probably extrapolate to variations in seeking help in managing menopause when induced by cancer too. In this chapter, the impact of cancer treatments on women from different ethnic backgrounds and health-seeking behaviour for problems caused by their cancer treatment, including menopause, will also be discussed.

Biological Differences between Different Ethnic Groups and the Experience of Menopausal Symptoms

The Study of Women's Health Across the Nation (SWAN) is a multi-site longitudinal cohort study in the United States of America which has been running since 1996 (1). The total numbers of women enrolled are relatively low (1,550 Caucasian, 935 African American, 286 Hispanic, 250 Chinese and 281 Japanese), and the study is limited in scope to women who are citizens of the United States of America. SWAN has nevertheless provided an invaluable insight into differences in hormonal fluctuations and symptom profiles between different ethnic groups.

When examining hormonal changes around the perimenopausal period, estradiol levels are shown to begin decreasing around two years prior to the final menstrual period and then continue decreasing for a further two years before plateauing. Follicle stimulating hormone (FSH) levels increase gradually, beginning seven years prior to the final menstrual period and accelerating two years prior to the final menstrual period. FSH levels continue to rise two years after the final menstrual period before levels stabilise (1). The timespan over which the changes in estradiol levels takes place appears to be shortened in women of Japanese and Chinese ethnicity compared to Caucasian and Afro-Caribbean women (1). The same data also suggests that obese women are less likely to experience a drop in estrogen levels and have a flatter trajectory of changes in estrogen and FSH, reflecting the altered estrogen production and storage in adipose tissue (6).

African and Caribbean

Women of African and Caribbean ethnicity were reported to have a longer duration of menopause transition with a greater proportion of anovulatory cycles compared to Caucasian women. The mean age of menopause for African American women is 49.6 (1, 7). Women from this ethnic background reported the highest prevalence, longest duration and greatest severity of vasomotor symptoms. They were also more likely to report shorter sleep duration, more frequent awakenings and poorer sleep quality. Weight gain and mental health issues associated with menopause were also prominently noted. Sexual function was noted to be of importance, and there was a smaller decline in sexual function compared to other groups. It was noted that women of African and Caribbean ethnicity may find it difficult to seek help from healthcare professionals regarding menopause symptoms despite the potential severity.

South-East Asian (Japan/China)

Women of Japanese or Chinese ethnicity were reported to experience longer menstrual cycles than Caucasian women during the perimenopausal period. The mean age of menopause in Japanese women is 48.3 (8). Women in this group were less likely to complain of severe vasomotor symptoms, but demonstrated a higher incidence of forgetfulness and joint and muscle pain. Sexual function was reported to be of less significance, and there was an increased incidence of loss of libido and dyspareunia. Women of Japanese and Chinese ethnicity had a lower bone mineral density compared to Caucasian women; however, their overall risk of osteoporotic fracture remained reduced despite this.

South Asian (India/Pakistan/Bangladesh/Sri Lanka)

The mean age of menopause in women of Indian ethnicity living in India is 46.7 years (9), and for Pakistani women, the mean age of menopause is 47.16 (10), reflecting a lower age across the Indian sub-continent than the quoted average of 51 in Western countries (11). The prevalence of premature ovarian insufficiency in this geographical region is reported at 1.5%, which is comparable to international rates (12). There is, however, a cultural tendency for women to have their families earlier in life, and so there may be an underreporting of premature ovarian insufficiency for women of south Asian ethnicity with concomitant impact on risk of cerebrovascular disease, dementia and osteoporosis in later life (13).

Women of south Asian ethnicity were more likely to raise concerns regarding vulval or urogynaecological symptoms (14) and less likely to discuss the impact of menopause on mental health than women from other cultural and ethnic backgrounds (15).

When assessing the evidence, however, this can sometimes be difficult to validate because the studies reporting on the experiences of women from ethnic minorities are from countries which are not their country of origin. The difficulty in seeking help may be related to language or cultural communication barriers or even prior experiences of being dismissed by healthcare professionals

Beliefs and Attitudes about Menopause

Cultural attitudes about menopause and its implications regarding the cessation of fertility vary widely around the world. The impact of the individual's ethnic background and pre-existing expectations must be viewed in the context of the culture in which the individual is living and the impact that has on their own personal cultural practices (14).

Menopause remains a taboo subject in many minority communities and is not always discussed openly, limiting women's ability to seek help from healthcare professionals (13). There may be a lack of awareness of symptoms and delayed diagnosis. There is usually a much lower uptake of HRT, and health inequalities may mean that women report a poorer experience of their menopause management which can be made worse when there are language barriers to communication.

The term for menopause in Arabic—'sinn al ya'—translates directly as 'the age of despair' (16), and in traditional cultures, the loss of childbearing status can represent a time of stress and uncertainty when women may fear being abandoned for a younger, more fertile woman (17). Whilst menopause can often be seen as an alteration of the women's role (13), it can also represent a freedom from the restrictions and taboos associated with menstruation (4). In some cultures menopausal women may take on the role of 'wise woman' status with an increased involvement in social, ritualistic and healing ceremonies (16). Guatemalan Mayan women are expected to enjoy increased freedom and status with menopause and the cessation of child rearing duties (18), and some traditional Irish Catholic women noted a sense of relief that their childbearing duties were behind them (19).

Other cultural groups such as South Asian women reported an overall neutral or positive outlook on menopause, although it was noted that the traditional and conservative nature of society acted as a potential barrier to seeking help from healthcare professionals (20).

The awareness of menopause as a part of the natural cycle of life can sometimes represent a barrier to women from different cultural backgrounds accessing healthcare because this can require challenging the predominant narrative of menopause as a natural event that does not require input from healthcare professionals (13, 21). Women from different cultural backgrounds may be more likely to opt for cultural or complementary medical therapies prior to seeking medical intervention (13). Chinese women may be more open to seeing a doctor and taking medication than other ethnic groups (14).

Health literacy can also pose a significant barrier to accessing services with language barriers and lack of representation posing a significant hurdle for some women from ethnic minority backgrounds.

Factors Contributing to Variation in Menopausal Experience

There are numerous factors associated with different cultural and ethnic backgrounds that can impact the symptoms associated with menopause. These can include but are not limited to diet, reproductive history, age of menarche, medical history, smoking history, BMI and previous use of oral contraceptives (3). Other factors that can influence women's experiences of these symptoms include the wider cultural implications of menopause and the cessation of childbearing and women's role in the wider community. Low socioeconomic status and unemployment are also known to be associated with a lower age at menopause (3).

The effect of socioeconomic status is powerful with data suggesting that women in lower socioeconomic groups are more likely to have significant vasomotor symptoms independent of cultural or ethnic background (22). Data from the USA suggests that the repeated activation of the stress response as attributed to persistent gender and racial discrimination causes a higher allostatic load on the body (23). This ongoing exposure to altered cortisol levels may have longer-term health implications (24) and greater impact on both the timing and experience of menopause (13).

Diet is often cited as potentially impacting menopausal symptoms, providing a non-medicalised method of modifying symptoms that women feel is within their control. Two of the most commonly discussed dietary modifications are the increased consumption of soy and other phytoestrogens and the Mediterranean diet.

The data surrounding the increased consumption of soy, either by dietary modification or nutritional supplements, is mixed. A systematic review showed that the increased consumption of soy isoflavone genistein as seen in the typical Japanese diet is associated with an overall reduction in vasomotor symptoms (25). Individual studies, however, show varying levels of impact on severity and frequency with increased dietary consumption with one study demonstrating no association between dietary intake of soy isoflavone genistein and vasomotor symptoms when confounding factors such as smoking are adjusted for (22). The increased consumption of soy isoflavone genistein is, however, positively associated with increased bone mineral density (26).

The impact of increased dietary intake of soy on breast cancer has also been a topic of debate with studies suggesting that phytoestrogens can have a negative impact on the treatment of hormone-sensitive breast cancers by reducing the efficacy of anti-oestrogenic medications (e.g. tamoxifen) (27). There is no clear consensus on the impact of increased dietary soy intake on the recurrence of breast cancer with some studies suggesting either a decreased risk (28) or no impact (29).

The Mediterranean diet is a diet characterised by a high intake of vegetables, legumes and whole grains and a lower intake of saturated animal fats. Overall, the diet is rich in polyphenols and omega-3 fatty acids with associated antioxidant and anti-inflammatory benefits (30). There have been suggestions that the Mediterranean diet is not only useful in managing obesity and the subsequent impact on cardiovascular risk factors but that it may also improve menopausal symptoms (30, 31). The significance of the Mediterranean diet in managing menopausal symptoms when its effects on weight loss are accounted for remains uncertain; however, given the known association between menopause and weight gain (27), any steps that women can take towards managing their BMI are likely to improve overall health.

Ethnic Variations in Response to Cancer Diagnosis and Health-Seeking Behaviour

An interesting variation of ethnicity and cancer diagnosis is that the overall incidence of cancer is lower in ethnic minorities (32) with a few exceptions including myeloma, Hodgkin's lymphoma, thyroid cancer and gastrointestinal cancers. In addition, studies have shown that there are ethnic variations in cancer symptom awareness and barriers to seeking help, with lowest levels observed in Bangladeshi and black Africans (5). These variations are poorly understood. This translates to more advanced disease at presentation, which is a key predictor of poor survival. The association of lower cancer awareness across all ethnic groups was noted with greater socioeconomic deprivation. This also indicates the association of levels of education to these indices.

An NHS England commissioned study undertaken to examine the lived experience of ethnic minority cancer patients in the UK identified several domains where experiences varied (33). These included the following:

i) Seeing GP and diagnostic tests: Participants felt that GPs did not always take their concerns and symptoms seriously, leading to misdiagnosis and late diagnosis resulting in a loss of trust in the healthcare system and seeking alternative routes to an accurate diagnosis.

ii) Getting a diagnosis: Cultural barriers to understanding and engaging with a diagnosis have been identified.

iii) Deciding the optimal treatment: Patients from ethnic minorities were less aware of treatment options, which made them feel forced into a decision.

iv) Difficulty accessing a clinical nurse specialist (nurses who are trained to provide expert care, advice and education to patients, families and fellow nursing staff): Patients from ethnic minorities described difficulties accessing a CNS as well as feeling isolated, unsupported and poorly informed about their cancer diagnosis.

v) Access to support groups: Barriers to accessing support groups which were appropriate to their cultural backgrounds were identified. This included support on discharge home.

vi) Care as an inpatient: Patients felt unable to ask questions when they were in hospital because they felt they were not listened to. There also appeared to be less continuity and lack of information on discharge.

It was also identified that in addition to ethnic groups these experiences varied based on other characteristics such as age, socioeconomic groups and disabilities. These variations have been identified across healthcare systems on both sides of the Atlantic (34).

The emotional distress caused by a cancer diagnosis in different ethnic groups also appears to be variable, with cancer survivors from ethnic minorities experiencing more distress than their white Caucasian counterparts. In a study conducted in the Netherlands, in which cancer-related variables were derived from the Netherlands Cancer Registry, survivors from South-Asian Surinamese, Moroccan, Turkish and Ghanaian origin reported more distress than survivors from Dutch origin (35).

When cancer results in an iatrogenic menopause, a variety of factors may therefore impact whether women seek help for these symptoms. These relate to healthcare provision, communication with healthcare providers and health-seeking behaviour based on cultural variations to the approach to menopause overall.

Summary

The Fawcett Society's 2022 report on Menopause and the Workplace identified differences in access to care and treatment in ethnic minorities (2). Aside from a delayed diagnosis (45% compared to 31% in white women), there were lower rates of HRT uptake (8% compared to 15% in white women). These differences in menopause care imply that women from ethnic minorities are being left out of conversations about menopause and its management. The experience of menopause can vary significantly between women from different cultural and ethnic backgrounds. Patterns of childrearing, socioeconomic status, diet and smoking status can all impact both the physical symptoms of menopause and the individual experience of the symptoms. Different cultural understandings of menopause can affect women's ability, or perception of their ability, to access healthcare treatment for their symptoms. Different diets are associated with potential impact on the symptoms of menopause experiences, most notably the positive impact of a diet high in soy on alleviating vasomotor symptoms and improving bone mineral density. The significance of this impact, though, is often difficult to disentangle from other factors such as smoking or BMI that also significantly impact overall health during the transitional period and into later life.

There is little if any research into the cultural variations of menopause care in women going through cancer treatment. In order to support women from ethnic minorities through a particularly difficult time in their lives when they are most vulnerable and going through treatment for a potentially life-threatening condition requires more research. There is a dire need to identify where these gaps in healthcare provision are so that they can be addressed and bridged appropriately.

References

1. Steinberg FM et al. Clinical outcomes of a 2-y soy isoflavone supplementation in menopausal women. Am J Clin Nutr. 2011 Feb;93(2):356–67.
2. Sabrina Keating on Behalf of the Wider WEAVE Team. Bridging the gap in menopause care for minority ethnic women. Nuffield Department of Primary Care Health Sciences. 2022.

Ref Type: Internet Communication

3. Amagai Y et al. Age at menopause and mortality in Japan: The Jichi Medical School Cohort Study. J Epidemiol. 2006 Jul;16(4):161–6.

4. Perna S et al. Multidimensional effects of soy isoflavone by food or supplements in menopause women: A systematic review and bibliometric analysis. Nat Prod Commun. 2016 Nov;11(11):1733–40.
5. Niksic M et al. Ethnic differences in cancer symptom awareness and barriers to seeking medical help in England. Br J Cancer. 2016 Jun 28;115(1):136–44.
6. Kriplani A, Banerjee K. An overview of age of onset of menopause in northern India. Maturitas. 2005 Nov;52(3–4):199–204.
7. Erdelyi A et al. The importance of nutrition in menopause and perimenopause-a review. Nutrients. 2023 Dec 21;16(1).
8. Robinson G. Cross-cultural perspectives on menopause. J Nerv Ment Dis. 1996 Aug;184(8):453–8.
9. BMS. Tool for clinicians what is the menopause? British Menopause Society. 2022.

Ref Type: Online Source

10. Nusrat N et al. Knowledge, attitude and experience of menopause. J Ayub Med Coll Abbottabad. 2008 Jan;20(1):56–9.
11. Pallikadavath S et al. Natural menopause among women below 50 years in India: A population-based study. Indian J Med Res. 2016 Sep;144(3):366–77.
12. Obermeyer CM. Menopause across cultures: A review of the evidence. Menopause. 2000 May;7(3):184–92.
13. Magee PJ, Rowland I. Soy products in the management of breast cancer. Curr Opin Clin Nutr Metab Care. 2012 Nov;15(6):586–91.
14. El Khoudary SR et al. The menopause transition and women's health at midlife: A progress report from the Study of Women's Health Across the Nation (SWAN). Menopause. 2019 Oct;26(10):1213–27.
15. Pugliese GD et al. Mediterranean diet as tool to manage obesity in menopause: A narrative review. Nutrition. 2020 Nov;79–80:110991.
16. Richardson LJ et al. Social status differences in allostatic load among young adults in the United States. SSM Popul Health. 2021 Sep;15:100771.
17. Vetrani C et al. Mediterranean diet: What are the consequences for menopause? Front Endocrinol (Lausanne). 2022;13:886824.
18. Mair KM et al. Obesity, estrogens and adipose tissue dysfunction—implications for pulmonary arterial hypertension. Pulm Circ. 2020 Jul;10(3):2045894020952019.
19. Shorey S, Ng ED. The experiences and needs of Asian women experiencing menopausal symptoms: A meta-synthesis. Menopause. 2019 May;26(5):557–69.
20. Melby MK et al. Culture and symptom reporting at menopause. Hum Reprod Update. 2005 Sep;11(5):495–512.
21. Prasad S. Menopause in ethnic minority women. Post Reprod Health. 2023 Dec;29(4):236–9.
22. Gold EB et al. Longitudinal analysis of the association between vasomotor symptoms and race/ethnicity across the menopausal transition: Study of Women's Health Across the Nation. Am J Public Health. 2006 Jul;96(7):1226–35.
23. Qazi RA. Age, pattern of menopause, climacteric symptoms and associated problems among urban population of Hyderabad, Pakistan. J Coll Physicians Surg Pak. 2006 Nov;16(11):700–3.
24. MacLellan J et al. Perimenopause and/or menopause help-seeking among women from ethnic minorities: A qualitative study of primary care practitioners' experiences. Br J Gen Pract. 2023 Jul;73(732):e511–18.
25. Inpan R et al. Isoflavone intervention and its impact on bone mineral density in postmenopausal women: A systematic review and meta-analysis of randomized controlled trials. Osteoporos Int. 2024 Mar;35(3):413–30.
26. Palmer JR et al. Onset of natural menopause in African American women. Am J Public Health. 2003 Feb;93(2):299–306.
27. Carolan M. Menopause: Irish women's voices. J Obstet Gynecol Neonatal Nurs. 2000 Jul;29(4):397–404.
28. Stewart DE. Menopause in highland Guatemala Mayan women. Maturitas. 2003 Apr 25;44(4):293–7.

29. Hall L et al. Meanings of menopause: Cultural influences on perception and management of menopause. J Holist Nurs. 2007 Jun;25(2):106–18.
30. Geronimus AT et al. "Weathering" and age patterns of allostatic load scores among blacks and whites in the United States. Am J Public Health. 2006 May;96(5):826–33.
31. Pitkin J. Cultural issues and the menopause. Menopause Int. 2010 Dec;16(4):156–61.
32. Delon C et al. Differences in cancer incidence by broad ethnic group in England, 2013–2017. Br J Cancer. 2022 Jun;126(12):1765–73.
33. The experiences of cancer patients from ethnic minority backgrounds in England: A qualitative study. NHS England Commissioned. 2020. Available from: https://northerncanceralliance.nhs.uk/wp-content/uploads/2021/09/NHSE-Qualitative-report-Experiences-of-ethnic-minority-patients-in-England-2020-1.pdf.

Ref Type: Internet Communication

34. Garrett E et al. Black cancer patients navigating a health-care system of racial discrimination. J Natl Cancer Inst. 2024 Feb 8;116(2):258–63.
35. Muller F et al. Emotional distress in cancer survivors from various ethnic backgrounds: Analysis of the multi-ethnic HELIUS study. Psychooncology. 2023 Sep;32(9):1412–23.

Chapter 3

Navigating Genetic Cancer Risk: Indications for Risk-Reducing Surgery and Managing Iatrogenic Menopause in Breast Cancer Patients

Darya Dahi and Jane Meisel

Clinical Scenario

Samantha is a 37-year-old G0P0 real estate agent who is engaged to be married. Her 41-year-old sister Kate was just diagnosed with node-positive, hormone receptor-positive (HR+) breast cancer, and underwent genetic testing that revealed a deleterious mutation in BRCA2. Samantha underwent testing as well and learned she had the same deleterious BRCA2 mutation. She is planning to undergo mammogram alternating with MRI for breast cancer screening for now, and is considering the option of prophylactic bilateral mastectomy for the future. However, she wonders about her risk for ovarian cancer; and as she embarks upon her marriage, asks what this means for her future fertility. How should you counsel her?

Introduction

Iatrogenic menopause is an important topic in breast cancer clinical practice and has become more pertinent in recent years. Patients with genetic mutations putting them at higher risk for breast and ovarian cancer often undergo bilateral salpingo-oophorectomy once they are finished with childbearing to reduce their ovarian cancer risk; and premenopausal patients with high-risk hormone receptor-positive (HR+) breast cancer benefit from ovarian suppression, whether surgical or

DOI: 10.1201/9781032631028-3

medical, to reduce their risk of cancer recurrence. The average American woman enters menopause in her early 50s, but these conditions often necessitate inducing menopause a decade (or more) earlier. Iatrogenic menopause is not without side effects, and many women struggle daily as a result of these challenges. In this chapter, we will focus on patients like Samantha, with deleterious mutations in *BRCA1* or *BRCA2,* and those with high-risk hormone receptor-positive (HR+) breast cancer, such as her sister Kate, who are recommended to undergo ovarian suppression, ablation, or removal to optimize their likelihood of breast cancer cure (in addition to the potential for ovarian cancer risk reduction). We will review the medical reasons that might necessitate induction of early menopause, explore the implications of this choice, and shed light on the evolving landscape of managing early menopause so that cancer risk can be optimally reduced while keeping quality of life at the forefront of the conversation.

BRCA Gene Mutations

Breast cancer is the most common cancer affecting women in the United States, with 310,720 predicted diagnoses in 2024 and an anticipated 42,250 deaths in 2024 alone (1). Ovarian cancer, on the other hand, has a much lower incidence rate but a greater mortality risk—data from the American Cancer Society demonstrates a 5-year survival rate of 91% for breast cancer, compared to a meager 51% for ovarian cancer (1). These statistics illustrate the critical need to understand risk factors to mitigate deaths and late-stage diagnoses.

The *BRCA* genes are tumor suppressor genes participating in the homologous recombination repair pathway. This pathway repairs double-strand DNA breaks, thus preventing excessive cell proliferation and preserving genome stability (2). Their status as the most important susceptibility genes associated with breast and ovarian cancer makes them the most extensively studied. Individuals carrying deleterious mutations in *BRCA1* have a lifetime risk of breast cancer (to age 80) ranging from 65% to 77%, while those with deleterious mutations in *BRCA2* have a lifetime risk ranging from 61% to 77% (3), compared to about 12% in the general population (4). For ovarian cancer, in a study that adjusted for patients who have not had a risk-reducing salpingo-oophorectomy (RRSO), ovarian cancer risk by age 70 can range from 38.8% to 57.9% for *BRCA1* carriers and 13.3% to 29.0% for *BRCA2* carriers (5). Because ovarian cancer is such a deadly disease and we do not have reliable methods for screening, RRSO is an important consideration for these patients. However, we do not want to induce menopause earlier than clinically necessary, or make fertility goals unnecessarily challenging to meet. Given these considerations, the timing of RRSO must be individualized to the greatest extent possible for each of our *BRCA* carrier patients.

Genetic Testing for BRCA

Following the identification of *BRCA1* and *BRCA2* mutations in breast and ovarian cancer patients in the 1990s (6), genetic testing became an important aspect of tailored and personalized cancer prevention and treatment for many individuals. Happily, accessibility of testing has improved significantly in the United States in the last ten years, due to legal and regulatory changes, guideline updates, and increased awareness. Until 2013, when the Supreme Court ruled against Myriad Genetics on the basis that natural phenomena may not be patented, BRCA mutation (BRCAm) screening tests were solely distributable by the molecular diagnostics company that had previously patented the *BRCA* genetic test (9). After this, other testing companies were able to enter the market, creating healthy competition and lowering testing costs, which in turn increased access to and supply of *BRCA* testing. Guidelines specifying the criteria for an individual to meet a recommendation for genetic testing have also changed since genetic testing was first made available. Recent NCCN guideline revisions have expanded testing criteria to allow for genetic testing for any patient diagnosed with breast cancer before age 65, or at any age in a patient for whom results could impact treatment decisions (7).

Revisions to extend indications for testing to include patients whose treatment plan could be changed by a positive result were brought about by the approval of *PARP* inhibitors in breast cancer, which first came about in the metastatic setting for patients with HER2-negative disease (10, 11). The OlympiAD trial (olaparib) and the EMBRACA trial (talazoparib) showed these drugs to be superior to chemotherapy in progression-free survival (PFS) as well as quality of life in patients with HER2-negative metastatic breast cancer who also had a deleterious *BRCA* mutation (10). These outcomes led to FDA (Food and Drug Administration) approval of these agents and guidelines from major international organizations recommending genetic testing for all patients with metastatic HER2-negative breast cancer (12). Later, when olaparib was approved as adjuvant therapy for *BRCA* mutation carriers with high-risk early-stage HER2-negative breast cancer, based on a trial that showed one year of adjuvant olaparib to reduce the risk of death from breast cancer in this population, genetic testing opportunities were expanded further (12).

These improvements in availability and accessibility of *BRCA* testing have resulted in increased genetic testing rates over time. A 2022 study looked at testing rates through the use of electronic health records and included over 200,000 women with documented *BRCA* testing results from 2007–2017 (8). The findings included an unsurprising but substantial increase in *BRCA* testing rates, with 34 in every 100,000 women in 2007 getting tested to 488 in every 100,000 in 2016 (8).

Now, patients like Kate, a premenopausal patient with node-positive, HR+ breast cancer, would likely be encouraged to undergo chemotherapy, breast surgery (bilateral mastectomy would be carefully considered, given her genetic mutation), as well as endocrine therapy, possibly including a CDK 4/6 inhibitor. In her case, bilateral salpingo-oophorectomy would serve as an important part of her endocrine therapy, as described in a later section of this manuscript, but also would prevent future ovarian cancer. Depending on the size of her tumor and number of positive nodes, Kate would also be a potential candidate for adjuvant olaparib. All of this treatment helps optimize patients' outcomes, but can also be overwhelming. In our clinical experience, we feel it is important to acknowledge the opportunity these advances provide for our patients, but also the challenges. Taking things one step at a time, and making sure patients know their team is there for them to help with side effect management and to empathize with their situation, can be of great comfort and value.

Recommendations Following a Positive *BRCAm* Test Result

When a patient tests positive for a deleterious *BRCA* mutation, even if, like Samantha, they do not have cancer, they still require counseling on several crucial health-related topics, including enhanced cancer screening protocols, risk-reducing surgeries, and fertility considerations, particularly for women who learn they are mutation carriers before they have had the chance to complete their families (13). Due to the lack of adequate early-detection screening techniques for ovarian cancer, women who are found to be *BRCAm* carriers are encouraged to contemplate RRSO, given that it is the most effective known method of reducing ovarian cancer risk (14).

RRSO is recommended after a patient has finished having children, but ideally between ages 35 and 40 for *BRCA1* mutation carriers and between ages 40 and 45 for *BRCA2* (14). For someone like Samantha, who is 37 and has a *BRCA2* mutation, having children before removing her ovaries seems appropriate, and we would recommend that the patient and her fiancé visit with a reproductive endocrinologist when they feel ready. This specialist can help them figure out a) whether, at advanced maternal age (over 35), she is likely to have difficulty conceiving naturally; and b) if they want to consider utilizing preimplantation genetic diagnosis to create and implant embryos that do not carry the deleterious *BRCA2* mutation. In addition, because inheriting two deleterious *BRCA2* mutations can cause severe Fanconi's anemia and other serious hematologic conditions that can result in premature loss of life, it will also be important for Samantha's fiancé to undergo genetic testing. Once Samantha has finished building her family, ideally before age 45, RRSO could be performed.

RRSO has been found to reduce the onset of ovarian malignancy by up to 96% (14), and given these success rates, it is performed frequently in mutation carriers—around 65% of female *BRCA1* mutation carriers are estimated to have RRSO before experiencing natural menopause (15). Inducing surgical menopause can save lives in women who are at the highest risk for ovarian cancer, but unfortunately, it can also have long-term, detrimental effects on heart health, bone health, metabolism, and quality of life (15). With rising rates of genetic testing, and hence, identification of *BRCAm* carriers, more individuals are enduring iatrogenic menopause for this reason. Consequently, the need to provide management options for challenges associated with early menopause has never been more relevant.

Iatrogenic Menopause for Breast Cancer

Iatrogenic menopause is not only employed as a preventative measure for ovarian cancer in patients with hereditary breast and ovarian cancer (HBOC) syndromes but, as referenced earlier, can be an important component of treatment for premenopausal women with high-risk hormone receptor-positive (HR+) breast cancer. Ovarian suppression in premenopausal breast cancer patients is often achieved medically (with injections of leuprolide, goserelin, or triptorelin) but sometimes is accomplished with oophorectomy. About 60% of premenopausal patients with breast cancer, like Kate in our clinical scenario, have HR+ disease (16). Many of these patients receive chemotherapy as well as endocrine therapy because premenopausal patients tend to have more aggressive tumor biology, but endocrine therapy remains the primary systemic treatment strategy for HR+ breast cancer. Advised endocrine therapies vary based on the menopausal status of the patient. Tamoxifen, a selective estrogen receptor modulator (SERM), is effective for both pre- and postmenopausal women because it prevents estrogen binding to receptors (17). Aromatase inhibitors (AIs) (e.g., anastrozole, exemestane, and letrozole) work to minimize circulating estrogen levels by hindering the transformation of androgen to estrogen. However, the use of aromatase inhibitors is limited to postmenopausal women because it does not decrease ovarian estrogen production (17).

AIs function by inhibiting the enzyme aromatase, which converts androgens into estrogens in various tissues including the fat cells and adrenal glands, which are where most estrogen production in postmenopausal women occurs (18). However, in premenopausal women, reducing endogenously synthesized estrogens via AIs may actually increase estrogen levels due to the negative feedback loop between the pituitary and gonads. When estrogen levels fall, the pituitary gland increases the secretion of gonadotropins, which stimulates the ovaries to produce more androgens and estrogens. This feedback mechanism can lead to an overall increase in circulating estrogen levels, rendering AIs ineffective in premenopausal women without concurrent ovarian suppression (18).

Following the publication of two randomized trials involving over 4,000 premenopausal women with HR+ breast cancer, the Suppression of Ovarian Function Trial (SOFT) and the Tamoxifen and Exemestane Trial (TEXT), the traditional approach of solely administering tamoxifen in premenopausal women was revised (16, 19). The two trials assigned women to either tamoxifen plus ovarian function suppression (OFS) or the AI exemestane plus OFS, with SOFT including a third arm of tamoxifen alone (16). In both trials, chemotherapy was optional. After an eight-year median follow-up, the SOFT study reported disease-free survival rates of 85.9% for patients treated with exemestane plus OFS and 83.2% for those treated with tamoxifen plus OFS. These rates are 7.0 and 4.2 percentage points higher, respectively, compared to the 78.9% rate of disease-free survival for patients treated with tamoxifen alone (16). The findings in SOFT support the efficacy of adding ovarian suppression to either form of adjuvant endocrine therapy in premenopausal women with sufficiently high-risk disease, and soon after these trials were initially reported, became a new standard of care. An analysis of the combined population in TEXT and SOFT whose regimen included OFS (>4,500 patients) reported an eight-year disease-free survival rate of 86.8% and 82.8% among patients assigned to receive exemestane and tamoxifen with OFS, respectively (16). The sustained higher rates for exemestane plus OFS provide some favorability towards the use of aromatase inhibitors over tamoxifen when paired with OFS, but also highlight that if AIs are not tolerated, tamoxifen + OFS is a viable option as well.

The findings from TEXT/SOFT have led to updates in numerous treatment protocols, including the ASCO (American Society of Clinical Oncology) Adjuvant Endocrine Therapy Guidelines. These now advise the use of OFS in conjunction with tamoxifen or aromatase inhibitors for women facing a higher risk of cancer recurrence (20). The criteria for identifying high-risk patients, while not definitively established, generally include those who would benefit from adjuvant chemotherapy (see Box 3.1).

BOX 3.1   BREAST CANCER PATIENTS IN WHOM OFS IS ADVISED

KEY RECOMMENDATIONS FOR OVARIAN SUPPRESSION

- STAGE II OR III: Women with stage II or III breast cancers, typically advised to undergo chemotherapy, should consider OFS alongside endocrine therapy.
- STAGE I OR II WITH HIGH RECURRENCE RISK: Women with stage I or II breast cancers at a higher risk of recurrence, in whom chemotherapy is a consideration, may also be offered OFS with endocrine therapy.
- CONTRAINDICATIONS: OFS is not recommended for women with stage I breast cancers that do not require chemotherapy or for those with node-negative cancers measuring 1 cm or less.

ADDITIONAL CONSIDERATIONS

- AGE ≤35 YEARS: Younger women (≤35 years) or those with involvement of four or more lymph nodes are particularly encouraged to include OFS as part of their treatment.
- CHEMOTHERAPY INDICATION: Patients with pathologically involved lymph nodes, large tumor size, high genomic risk of recurrence, or other high-risk features who have received chemotherapy.
- LOW-RISK PATIENTS: Tamoxifen alone remains the standard for women at low risk of relapse, as defined by clinical, immunohistochemical, and genomic parameters.

Decisions about adjuvant systemic treatment, including OFS, should be driven by the extent of disease, tumor biology, and patient comorbidities. While formal high-risk criteria are ill-defined, younger age at diagnosis or the presence of factors warranting chemotherapy merit careful consideration of the inclusion of OFS in the treatment regimen. Nonetheless, the benefits of OFS must be carefully weighed with the risks of both short-term and longer-term adverse effects.

Ovarian Function Suppression: Different Techniques

OFS, by definition, causes premature menopause, which leads to a greater risk of low bone density (21), which can be associated with increased fracture incidence, elevated risk of coronary artery disease (22), increased cardiovascular mortality, and overall mortality (22, 23). Additionally, studies have shown that women with premature ovarian failure (POF) experience decreased overall physical and sexual health and lower levels of satisfaction with their sexual lives (24). Mental health is another crucial aspect affected by premature ovarian failure, something we see anecdotally in our patients who enter menopause earlier than anticipated, but also in small but notable reports in the published literature. One in particular reporting on 81 women who experienced POF (unrelated to cancer) and compared to controls showed that POF increases anxiety, depression, and psychological distress (24). Such adverse effects associated with early menopause require careful consideration with any patient considering ovarian suppression—surgical or medical— since these kinds of cost-benefit evaluations are intrinsically personal.

Kwon et al. created the Markov Monte Carlo simulation model to estimate the costs and benefits of different endocrine strategies for premenopausal women with ER+ early breast cancer. The model compared three treatment options: tamoxifen alone, medical ovarian ablation alongside an AI regimen, and surgical ovarian ablation alongside an AI regimen (25). The model was primarily used to measure incremental cost-effectiveness ratio (ICER), defined as the additional cost divided by the incremental health benefit compared to an alternative treatment option. A treatment with less than $100,000 per year of life gained was considered cost-effective. The model found that tamoxifen alone was the ideal strategy for women at a low risk of recurrence (a subgroup without chemotherapy), with the highest life expectancy gain at the lowest cost (25). For women at high risk, the BSO group yielded a higher average life expectancy at an acceptable cost (16.78 years, $25,368) relative to tamoxifen alone (16.55 years, $1,523), with an ICER of $102,290. GnRHa-AI was more effective (yielding the highest average life expectancy) but appreciably pricier (16.93 years, $91,170), with an ICER of $443,375 (25). The results of this study demonstrate better cost-effectiveness for BSO compared to medical ovarian suppression for higher-risk ER+ breast cancer patients; however, they also emphasize the heavily personal considerations that must be considered with ovarian ablation.

Both routes of ovarian suppression result in early menopause and, as mentioned previously, are correlated with various adverse effects. However, these routes have been demonstrated to reduce all-cause mortality in *BRCAm* carriers (26, 27), making ovarian suppression justifiable in such populations. Additionally, a small minority of these women (those with HR- cancers who have had bilateral mastectomies) have the option to manage adverse effects and downstream health risks with hormone replacement therapies (HRT) (28), which are contraindicated in HR+ breast cancer (23).

The largest distinction in ovarian ablation by BSO and medical OFS lies in reversibility. BSO causes irreversible ovarian suppression, while the use of GnRH agonists makes for a reversible method of achieving ovarian suppression (29). With BSO, ablation cannot be undone to reduce side effects, while with GnRH agonists, cessation of medication will allow for a reversal in suppression with an expectancy that side effects can diminish. The reversibility of GnRH agonists was supported by a Zoladex Early Breast Cancer Research Association study that evaluated the tolerability of the GnRH agonist goserelin. Once goserelin therapy stopped, menses returned in 90% of amenorrheic breast cancer patients under the age of 40 and in 70% of those above the age of 40 (30, 31). Age is often an important consideration in patients with HR+ breast cancer when contemplating options for ovarian suppression. The SOFT and TEXT trials only studied five years of ovarian suppression, and more than that can be hard for patients to tolerate. If a woman is 48 years old and premenopausal at the time of a higher-risk HR+ breast cancer diagnosis, BSO may be a very reasonable option because, by the time she is 53, it is likely she may be in natural menopause already. But if the same woman is 35 at the time of diagnosis and would be only 40 by the end of her five years of ovarian suppression, permanent ovarian suppression may come at considerable personal cost. This may be someone for whom GnRH agonists are more appropriate.

Clinical Scenario

Four years later, Samantha is 41 years old and after discussion with a reproductive endocrinologist, opted to conceive naturally with her husband (who was tested and found to be BRCA2 negative). She had a healthy baby at 39 years of age and nursed for 12 months, and is now contemplating bilateral mastectomy. She and her husband feel their family is complete with one child, and she is starting to contemplate timing of BSO as well.

Kate has completed surgery, chemotherapy, and radiation. She was not a candidate for adjuvant olaparib because she only had two positive nodes, but she had a BSO and completed two years of aromatase inhibitor therapy plus abemaciclib and is now on an aromatase inhibitor alone. She has been experiencing hot flashes and depressive symptoms. How would you counsel her?

Managing Ovarian Suppression by Symptom

Vasomotor symptoms (such as hot flashes and sweating), vaginal atrophy, and sleep disturbances are unpleasant side effects of menopause that can deeply affect everyday life. Addressing these symptoms presents a complex task. Because hormone replacement therapy (HRT) is contraindicated for women with HR+ breast carcinoma or those at increased risk for this, the quest for alternative approaches becomes imperative. This section explores pharmacological and non-pharmacological interventions tailored to address the diverse associated symptoms of ovarian suppression.

Vasomotor Symptoms

Vasomotor symptoms (VMS), particularly hot flashes, represent a significant challenge for women undergoing breast cancer treatment, often impacting their quality of life (QoL) and treatment adherence. Estrogen suppression disrupts the hypothalamic perception of core body temperature, leading to the onset of hot flashes (32). These are prevalent among women receiving endocrine therapy, with reports indicating their occurrence in up to 80% of patients on tamoxifen and up to 93% with the addition of OFS (33). Notably, younger patients tend to experience more severe symptoms, exacerbating the negative effects on QoL (33, 34).

Effective management strategies for VMS are crucial. With regard to non-pharmacological interventions, cognitive behavioral therapy (CBT) has shown promise in randomized trials, including a Phase III nurse-led group CBT trial (35, 36). In the nurse-led group CBT trial, participants were divided into two cohorts: group CBT and usual care. The trial found a statistically significant difference between the groups after 26 weeks, finding that the women's problem ratings for hot flashes and night sweats experienced a reduction by 46% in the CBT group and only a 15% reduction in the usual care group (36). Additional benefits of the group CBT included a decreased frequency of hot flashes and night sweats, enhanced sleep quality, diminished levels of anxiety and depression, and less disruption to daily activities (36). The use of acupuncture to manage vasomotor symptoms in women going through menopause is a contentious topic. While some trials suggest acupuncture can reduce symptoms like hot flashes (37–39), the evidence remains mixed. A systematic review of trials on acupuncture for menopause suggests that acupuncture shows effectiveness when there is no alternative treatment; however, its efficacy is not superior to that of sham treatments (40). The complexity of acupuncture as a treatment, the physiological effects of sham acupuncture, and the placebo phenomenon all contribute to the ambiguity of trial results (41). The debate is further fueled by the variety of control treatments used in different studies, including sham acupuncture, hormone therapy, and applied relaxation, making it difficult to assess acupuncture's relative effectiveness. While the evidence is not uniformly persuasive across all studies, there is a general trend indicating acupuncture's beneficial impact, particularly in contrast with no intervention at all. Coupled with its safety and minimal side effects, the potential benefits of acupuncture likely outweigh the risks, making it a worthwhile consideration for the management of vasomotor symptoms (40). Where available, we recommend offering acupuncture to breast cancer patients, particularly those who desire non-pharmacologic interventions for menopausal symptoms. We make sure patients know that if they opt to try acupuncture and it becomes costly or inconvenient, or is not effective, they can always stop.

As for non-hormonal pharmacological interventions, clonidine is a centrally acting α-adrenergic agonist that increases the sweating threshold by lowering the release of norepinephrine (41). One trial looking at clonidine via a transdermal patch versus placebo in 110 women with a history of breast carcinoma showed that the clonidine group had a 20% reduction in hot flashes as compared to the placebo group (42). However, despite the relief provided by clonidine, it is often not recommended unless symptoms are highly refractory to other remedies due to the numerous side effects found in trials, including mouth dryness, itching, drowsiness, and difficulty sleeping (43).

Selective serotonin reuptake inhibitors and selective norepinephrine reuptake inhibitors (SSRIs/SNRIs) are other pharmacological agents that have been shown to relieve hot flashes on top of their function as antidepressants and are commonly used in clinical practice (44, 45). They are neurotransmitter modulators found in a quantitative comparison to lessen the frequency of hot flashes by 1.2–1.7 times per day more than the placebo (44). However, there can be effects associated with the central nervous system, namely, insomnia, nausea, dry mouth, dizziness, and anxiety (44, 46). Notable, also, are symptoms of sexual dysfunction, such as hypoactive desire and orgasm dysfunction, found in some studies to be prevalent in up to 80% of women taking antidepressants (47).

There has historically been concern that some SSRIs and SNRIs may reduce the efficacy of tamoxifen, particularly those that are inhibitors of CYP2D6, which tamoxifen requires in order to be metabolized into endoxifen, its active form. One cohort study analyzed data from women who were co-prescribed an SSRI (either paroxetine, fluoxetine, sertraline, citalopram, or fluvoxamine) or venlafaxine (an SSRI and an SSNI) with tamoxifen treatment and looked at whether co-prescriptions affected the risk of death from breast cancer. The study found that paroxetine use was associated with an elevated risk of death from breast cancer, but that exposure to the other SSRIs during tamoxifen treatment did not show an increased risk of breast cancer mortality (48). However, later studies have not confirmed this association (49, 50). Given the inconclusive nature of the evidence, the practice of many breast oncologists is to prioritize SSRIs with lower levels of CYP2D6 inhibition (such as sertraline and citalopram) when prescribing these medications to patients on tamoxifen, but not to absolutely require a patient to stop paroxetine or other SSRIs/SNRIs if they rely on these medications to support their mental health. Finally, another comprehensive literature evaluation found that venlafaxine and duloxetine have greater efficacy in reducing the frequency and severity of hot flashes compared to other SSRIs/SNRIs in breast cancer patients (51). Venlafaxine is a weak inhibitor of CYP2D6, thereby having less of an effect on tamoxifen; so this is often a good medication to start with in patients who experience hot flashes and mood changes after starting tamoxifen therapy.

Along with SSRIs and SNRIs, evidence-based clinical recommendations published in 2015 by the Endocrine Society's Menopause Task Force suggest gabapentin or pregabalin for women seeking non-hormonal pharmacological management for moderate to severe vasomotor symptoms (52). Gabapentin and pregabalin are both medications that belong to the class of drugs known as gabapentinoids (53). Gabapentin has gained recognition as a significant nonhormonal alternative for the management of vasomotor symptoms, such as hot flashes, in menopausal women. Initially identified as a potential treatment in a case series report, gabapentin's efficacy was subsequently supported by two pilot trials (54–56). These early studies paved the way for more rigorous investigations into its therapeutic benefits, including a placebo-controlled trial involving 59 postmenopausal women, which revealed that a daily dose of 900 mg of gabapentin led to a 45% reduction in hot flash frequency and a 54% decrease in overall hot flash scores after 12 weeks of treatment. These outcomes were significantly superior to those observed with the placebo group, which only achieved reductions of 29% and 31%, respectively (57). However, gabapentin was associated with side effects such as somnolence and dizziness. Further evidence of gabapentin's effectiveness came from another randomized, placebo-controlled trial with 420 breast cancer patients. The study demonstrated that gabapentin, administered at 100 mg three times per day, reduced hot flash scores by 31%, while a higher dose of 300 mg three times per day achieved a 46% reduction (P = 0.007) (58). More recent studies have continued to validate gabapentin's utility. While its use comes with potential side effects, these investigations underscore gabapentin's role as an efficacious nonhormonal agent for hot flash management.

Oxybutynin has recently emerged as an effective and well-tolerated intervention for reducing vasomotor symptoms and improving quality-of-life measures (43). Oxybutynin is an FDA-approved anticholinergic drug for the treatment of overactive bladder symptoms. Unlike many SSRIs and SNRIs, oxybutynin is not significantly metabolized by CYP2D6 and, thus, has no interference with CYP2D6, giving it an advantage for those on a tamoxifen regimen (59). A randomized trial studying the effects of oxybutynin included women both with and without breast cancer and found alleviation of hot flashes in both frequency and severity. Its positive impact on measures of hot flash interference and quality of life was clinically significant and even surpassed reductions observed with antidepressants, making it a promising option for women who are not candidates for HRT (59).

Clinical Scenario

Three years later, Kate is doing much better. She completed her five years of endocrine therapy and has opted for extended adjuvant endocrine therapy to reduce her risk of recurrence further, given her positive nodes. She found acupuncture to be helpful for hot flash management, and also started on venlafaxine in the hopes that it would improve her mood as well. She joined a support group for breast cancer patients and found a good therapist, and the combination of these interventions made her feel "like my old self again." She became busy with work and other commitments, and eventually stopped the acupuncture because of her schedule, but she feels comfortable without it. However, she now has vaginal dryness, which has impacted her intimacy with her husband.

Samantha underwent bilateral mastectomies at age 42, and one year later, underwent BSO. She felt emotionally overwhelmed afterwards, and at Kate's encouragement, started seeing a therapist, which helped greatly. She has her first bone density test (suggested by her primary care doctor because she is now in menopause and is a small-boned, Caucasian woman) and to her surprise, is found to have osteoporosis.

How would you counsel the sisters now?

Genitourinary Syndrome of Menopause or Vaginal Dryness and Atrophy

The term *genitourinary syndrome of menopause* (GSM) is defined by the American College of Obstetricians and Gynecologists (ACOG) as "a constellation of symptoms that relate to hypoestrogenic effects on the genital epithelium, such as genital dryness, burning, and irritation; potential downstream effects of vulvar and vaginal atrophy such as dyspareunia; urinary symptoms such as urgency or dysuria; and recurrent urinary tract infections" (60). Reduced estrogen levels, particularly affecting urinary and vaginal receptors, can have adverse effects such as atrophic vaginitis—experienced by many during menopause. This condition afflicts nearly 70% of postmenopausal breast cancer survivors as opposed to 50% of postmenopausal women without a history of breast cancer, warranting special attention to management options in this population (61, 62). For Kate, who is not a candidate for hormone replacement given that she has had a node-positive, HR+ breast cancer, this is particularly challenging.

The American College of Obstetrics and Gynecology (ACOG) has published consensus recommendations for the management of GSM among women with HR+ breast cancers (see Box 3.2) (60).

BOX 3.2   ACOG RECOMMENDATIONS FOR MANAGEMENT OF VAGINAL ATROPHY

1. Primary consideration should be given to nonhormonal approaches for managing urogenital symptoms in individuals with a background of estrogen-dependent breast cancer.
2. Familiarity with the various nonhormonal treatment options is necessary, since trials of numerous options may be necessary to identify effective treatment for each patient.
3. Nonhormonal treatments reported as effective in alleviating vulvovaginal symptoms include silicone-, polycarbophil-, and water-based lubricants; hyaluronic acid; polyacrylic acid; and vaginal suppositories containing vitamin E and D. Superiority of one approach over the others is not made possible due to insufficient data.

Clinical trial findings for a polycarbophil-based vaginal moisturizer indicate enhancements in vaginal dryness, dyspareunia, sexual satisfaction and frequency, and vaginal pH when used regularly (two to three times per week) (63). There are a variety of vaginal moisturizers that may relieve vulvovaginal symptoms, though prioritization should be given to those supposed by evidence of efficacy and that are pH-balancing. Extended use is crucial, because it may take one to three months to observe significant results (64).

Clinical Scenario

Kate begins using a vaginal moisturizer every three days, and a lubricant prior to sexual activity. She is aware that once she finishes her course of aromatase inhibitor therapy, which brings her estrogen levels even lower than they typically would be in menopause, this may improve somewhat. In the meantime, she finds that her osteopenia, which was present on her bone density test two years ago, has worsened to the point of osteoporosis. She and Samantha together start looking into options to optimize bone health.

Bone Health

The administration of GnRH agonists for ovarian suppression, surgical oophorectomy, or the onset of early menopause due to chemotherapy significantly diminishes circulating estrogen levels. This hormonal reduction precipitates an accelerated rate of bone resorption, leading to a marked decrease in bone mineral density (BMD). The most substantial reduction in BMD is typically observed within the first year of treatment (65). Research has quantified this loss, showing an average annual decrease in total body BMD of approximately 5% with the use of GnRH agonists (66). Furthermore, studies have recorded a dramatic decline of 18% to 19% in BMD over a span of two years following oophorectomy (67). Premenopausal breast cancer patients who receive OFS, particularly with AIs, are at a heightened risk for significant bone loss and must monitor their BMD (68). In premenopausal women with breast cancer who underwent two years of OFS, there was an overall 10.5% reduction in bone mineral density at the lumbar spine and a 6.4% reduction at the femoral neck (69). These findings underscore the profound impact such treatments have on skeletal health.

Lifestyle changes, including dietary and physical accommodations, are among the simplest and most relevant prevention tactics for bone density reduction. ASCO Clinical Practice Guidelines assert that all patients with or at risk of osteoporosis should be encouraged to consume a diet with adequate calcium and vitamin D. An intake of 1,000 to 1,200 mg/d of calcium and 800 to 1,000 IU/d of vitamin D is recommended, whether through the use of food sources or supplements (70). Regular physical activity should also be encouraged, since exercise serves as an effective intervention for improving a multitude of side effects experienced by breast cancer patients, including but not limited to cognitive impairment, depression, pain, cardiopulmonary function, and bone density (71). Resistance exercise (achieved through resistance bands or weights) has been shown to improve bone density and QoL when performed during and following cancer treatment (72, 73).

Pharmacological strategies to counteract bone density loss in breast cancer patients have shown promising results, particularly with the use of bisphosphonates. Meta-analyses, such as the one conducted by the Early Breast Cancer Trialists' Collaborative Group, which included over 18,000 patients, have highlighted the efficacy of bisphosphonates like zoledronic acid and ibandronic acid. The treatment, lasting an average of 3.4 years, significantly decreased the occurrence of bone metastases and breast cancer mortality in postmenopausal individuals. Current guidelines suggest considering adjuvant bisphosphonate therapy for all postmenopausal patients with primary breast cancer (74). Zoledronic acid is often the first choice due to its robust clinical backing and lower discontinuation rates due to side effects (75). Moreover, the AZURE trial reported a significant reduction in the five-year fracture rate among women receiving adjuvant zoledronate during anti-estrogen therapy (76).

Clinical Scenario

Both sisters start receiving zoledronic acid every six months, and taking vitamin D daily. They also embark upon a walking program four days per week, which they find enhances their mental health and their sleep. Kate loses five pounds over the course of four months, which makes her pleased because she has gained several unwanted pounds while on endocrine therapy. Two years later, both of their bone density tests are improved.

Conclusion

Managing OFS-induced symptoms presents a multifaceted challenge, particularly in breast cancer patients in whom traditional HRT is contraindicated. These symptoms, ranging from vasomotor disruptions to genitourinary discomfort, significantly impact patients' quality of life and treatment adherence. In the collective data from the SOFT and TEXT studies, 19% of patients ceased ovarian suppression treatment with the GnRH agonist triptorelin prematurely, without replacing it with ovarian ablation (15). Among breast cancer patients, non-adherence to and premature termination of endocrine therapy regimens are associated with diminished overall survival outcomes (77). Hence, the management of iatrogenic menopausal symptoms is a vital component of clinical breast oncology.

It should be noted that many secondary symptoms associated with menopause, such as sleep disturbances, mental health, and changes in sexual drive, may be intertwined with vasomotor or genitourinary syndrome of menopause (GSM) symptoms. Hence, like in Kate's case, addressing one symptom (hot flashes) may also lead to improvements in other areas that impact her quality of life (sleep, mood). Nonhormonal interventions play a crucial role in symptom management, offering relief without the risk of hormone-related complications. Cognitive behavioral therapy, nonhormonal pharmacological agents like oxybutynin and SSRIs, and various vaginal moisturizers have shown promise in alleviating symptoms and improving quality of life. Breast care specialists should remain vigilant in exploring and offering these diverse treatment options to ensure comprehensive and tailored care for breast cancer patients experiencing ovarian suppression-induced symptoms.

Summary

With advancements in medical science allowing for greater numbers of women undergoing *BRCA* testing and allowing us to treat many breast cancer patients more effectively by putting them into biochemical menopause, the significance of minimizing the adverse effects associated with lack of ovarian function is becoming increasingly pronounced. Healthcare providers and patients alike must strive to find comprehensive approaches that address not only the immediate concerns but also the long-term consequences of altered hormonal landscapes. Further research into the efficacy and safety of existing nonhormonal interventions is warranted. Collaborative efforts between clinicians and researchers are essential to identify and implement optimal management strategies that optimize both quality of life and treatment outcomes for this patient population.

References

1. Siegel RL et al. Cancer statistics, 2024. CA Cancer J Clin. 2024;74(1):12–49.
2. Venkitaraman AR. Functions of BRCA1 and BRCA2 in the biological response to DNA damage. J Cell Sci. 2001;114(20):3591–8.

3. Chen S, Parmigiani G. Meta-analysis of BRCA1 and BRCA2 penetrance. J Clin Oncol. 2007;25(11):1329.
4. Kuchenbaecker KB et al. Risks of breast, ovarian, and contralateral breast cancer for BRCA1 and BRCA2 mutation carriers. JAMA. 2017;317(23):2402.
5. Chen J et al. Penetrance of breast and ovarian cancer in women who carry a BRCA1/2 mutation and do not use risk-reducing salpingo-oophorectomy: An updated meta-analysis. JNCI Cancer Spectr. 2020;4(4):pkaa029.
6. Daly MB et al. NCCN guidelines insights: Genetic/familial high-risk assessment: Breast, ovarian, and pancreatic, version 1.2020: Featured updates to the NCCN guidelines. J Natl Compr Canc Netw. 2020;18(4):380–91.
7. National Comprehensive Cancer Network. Genetic/familial high-risk assessment: Breast, ovarian, and pancreatic, version 1.2020. J Natl Comp Cancer Netw. 2020;18(4):380–91.
8. Bedrosian I et al. Germline testing in patients with breast cancer: ASCO-society of surgical oncology guideline. J Clin Oncol. 2024;42(5):584.
9. Klutsky T, Weinmeyer R. Supreme court to myriad genetics: Synthetic DNA is patentable but isolated genes are not. AMA J Ethics. 2015;17(9):849–53.
10. Litton JK et al. Talazoparib in patients with advanced breast cancer and a germline BRCA mutation. New Engl J Med. 2018;379(8):753–63.
11. Tung N, Garber JE. PARP inhibition in breast cancer: Progress made and future hopes. NPJ Breast Cancer. 2022;8(1):47.
12. Paluch-Shimon S et al. Prevention and screening in BRCA mutation carriers and other breast/ovarian hereditary cancer syndromes: ESMO Clinical Practice Guidelines for cancer prevention and screening. Ann Oncol. 2016;27(5_suppl):v103–10.
13. Tutt ANJ et al. Adjuvant olaparib for patients with BRCA1- or BRCA2-mutated breast cancer. N Engl J Med. 2021;384(25):2394.
14. Gasparri ML et al. Risk-reducing bilateral salpingo-oophorectomy for BRCA mutation carriers and hormonal replacement therapy: If it should rain, better a drizzle than a storm. Medicina. 2019;55(8).
15. Francis PA et al. Tailoring adjuvant endocrine therapy for premenopausal breast cancer. New Engl J Med. 2018;379(2):122.
16. Kotsopoulos J et al. Hormone replacement therapy after oophorectomy and breast cancer risk among BRCA1 mutation carriers. JAMA Oncol. 2018;4(8):1059–66.
17. Wirk B. The role of ovarian ablation in the management of breast cancer. Breast J. 2005;11(6):416–24.
18. Miller WR. Aromatase inhibitors: Mechanism of action and role in the treatment of breast cancer. Seminars Oncol. 2023;30:3–11.
19. Oseledchyk A et al. Surgical ovarian suppression for adjuvant treatment in hormone receptor positive breast cancer in premenopausal patients. Int J Gynecol Cancer. 2021;31(2):222.
20. Burstein HJ et al. Adjuvant endocrine therapy for women with hormone receptor-positive breast cancer: American Society of Clinical Oncology clinical practice guideline update on ovarian suppression. J Clin Oncol. 2016;34(14):1689–701.
21. Gallagher JC. Effect of early menopause on bone mineral density and fractures. Menopause. 2007;14(3 Pt 2):567–71.
22. Mondul AM et al. Age at natural menopause and cause-specific mortality. Am J Epidemiol. 2005;62(11):1089–97.
23. Khan F et al. Oophorectomy in premenopausal patients with estrogen receptor-positive breast cancer: New insights into long-term effects. Current Oncol. 2023;30(2):1794–804.
24. Van der Stege JG et al. Decreased androgen concentrations and diminished general and sexual well-being in women with premature ovarian failure. Menopause. 2008;15(1):23–31.
25. Kwon JS et al. Long-term consequences of ovarian ablation for premenopausal breast cancer. Breast Cancer Res Treat. 2016;157(3):565–73.
26. Domchek SM et al. Association of risk-reducing surgery in BRCA1 or BRCA2 mutation carriers with cancer risk and mortality. JAMA. 2010;304(9):967.
27. Finch PM et al. Impact of oophorectomy on cancer incidence and mortality in women with a BRCA1 or BRCA2 mutation. J Clin Oncol. 2014;32(15):1547–53.

28. Rebbeck TR et al. Effect of short-term hormone replacement therapy on breast cancer risk reduction after bilateral prophylactic oophorectomy in BRCA1 and BRCA2 mutation carriers: The PROSE Study Group. J Clin Oncol. 2005;23(31):7804–10.

29. Jiang M et al. Adjuvant ovarian suppression for premenopausal hormone receptor-positive breast cancer: A network meta-analysis. Medicine. 2021;100(33).

30. Jonat W et al. Goserelin versus cyclophosphamide, methotrexate, and fluorouracil as adjuvant therapy in premenopausal patients with node-positive breast cancer: The Zoladex Early Breast Cancer Research Association Study. J Clin Oncol. 2002;20(24):4628–35.

31. Haes H et al. Quality of life in goserelin-treated versus cyclophosphamide + methotrexate + fluorouracil-treated premenopausal and perimenopausal patients with node-positive, early breast cancer: The Zoladex Early Breast Cancer Research Association Trialists Group. J Clin Oncol. 2003;21(24):4510–16.

32. Lambertini M et al. Advances in the management of menopausal symptoms, fertility preservation, and bone health for women with breast cancer on endocrine therapy. Am Soc Clin Oncol Educ Book (ASCO Annual Meeting). 2023;43:e390442.

33. Franzoi MA et al. Evidence-based approaches for the management of side-effects of adjuvant endocrine therapy in patients with breast cancer. Lancet Oncol. 2021;22(7):e303–13.

34. Carpenter JS et al. Hot flashes in postmenopausal women treated for breast carcinoma. Cancer. 1998;82(9):1682–91.

35. Mann E et al. Cognitive behavioral treatment for women who have menopausal symptoms after breast cancer treatment (MENOS 1): A randomised controlled trial. Lancet Oncol. 2012;13(3): 309–18.

36. Fenlon D et al. Effectiveness of nurse-led group CBT for hot flushes and night sweats in women with breast cancer: Results of the MENOS4 randomised controlled trial. Psycho-Oncol. 2020; 29(10):1514–23.

37. Hervik J, Mjåland O. Acupuncture for the treatment of hot flashes in breast cancer patients, a randomized, controlled trial. Breast Cancer Res Treat. 2009;116(2):311–16.

38. Bokmand S, Flyger H. Acupuncture relieves menopausal discomfort in breast cancer patients: A prospective, double blinded, randomized study. Breast. 2013;22(3):320–3.

39. Frisk J et al. Acupuncture improves Health-Related Quality-of-Life (HRQoL) and sleep in women with breast cancer and hot flushes. Support Care Cancer. 2012;20(4):715–24.

40. Ee C et al. Acupuncture for menopausal hot flashes: Clinical evidence update and its relevance to decision making. Menopause. 2017;24(8):980–7.

41. Freedman RR, Dinsay R. Clonidine raises the sweating threshold in symptomatic but not in asymptomatic postmenopausal women. Fertil Steril. 2000;74(1):20–3.

42. Goldberg RM et al. Transdermal clonidine for ameliorating tamoxifen-induced hot flashes. J Clin Oncol. 1994;12(1):155–8.

43. Pachman DR. Management of menopause-associated vasomotor symptoms: Current treatment options, challenges and future directions. Int J Women's Health. 2010;2:123–35.

44. Li T et al. Quantitative comparison of drug efficacy in treating hot flashes in patients with breast cancer. Breast Cancer Res Treat. 2019;173(3):511–20.

45. Fenlon D et al. Management of hot flushes in UK breast cancer patients: Clinician and patient perspectives. J Psychosom Obstet Gynecol. 2017;38(4):276–83.

46. Leon-Ferre RA. Management of hot flashes in women with breast cancer receiving ovarian function suppression. Cancer Treat Rev. 2017;52:82–90.

47. La Torre A et al. Sexual dysfunction related to psychotropic drugs: A critical review—part I: Antidepressants. Pharmacopsychiatry. 2013;46(5):191–9.

48. Kelly CM et al. Selective serotonin reuptake inhibitors and breast cancer mortality in women receiving tamoxifen: A population based cohort study. BMJ. 2010;340.

49. Busby J et al. Selective serotonin reuptake inhibitor use and breast cancer survival: A population-based cohort study. Breast Cancer Res. 2018;20(1):4.

50. Donneyong MM et al. Risk of mortality with concomitant use of tamoxifen and selective serotonin reuptake inhibitors: Multi-database cohort study, BMJ. 2016;354:i5014.
51. Stubbs C et al. Do SSRIs and SNRIs reduce the frequency and/or severity of hot flashes in menopausal women. J Oklahoma State Med Assoc. 2017;110(5):272.
52. Stuenkel CA et al. Treatment of symptoms of the menopause: An endocrine society clinical practice guideline. J Clin Endocrinol Metab. 2015;100(11):3975–4011.
53. Chincholkar M. Gabapentinoids: Pharmacokinetics, pharmacodynamics and considerations for clinical practice. Br J Pain. 2020;14(2):104–14.
54. Guttuso TJ. Gabapentin's effects on hot flashes and hypothermia. Neurol. 2000;54(11):2161–3.
55. Loprinzi L et al. Pilot evaluation of gabapentin for treating hot flashes. Mayo Clin Proc. 2002;77(11):1159–63.
56. Pandya KJ et al. Pilot study using gabapentin for tamoxifen-induced hot flashes in women with breast cancer. Breast Cancer Res Treat. 2004;83(1):87–9.
57. Guttuso T et al. Gabapentin's effects on hot flashes in postmenopausal women: A randomized controlled trial. Obstet Gynecol. 2003;101(2):337–45.
58. Pandya KJ et al. Gabapentin for hot flashes in 420 women with breast cancer: A randomised double-blind placebo-controlled trial. Lancet. 2005;366(9488):818–24.
59. Leon-Ferre RA et al. Oxybutynin vs Placebo for hot flashes in women with or without breast cancer: A randomized, double-blind clinical trial (ACCRU SC-1603). JNCI Cancer Spectr. 2020; 4(1):pkz088.
60. Treatment of urogenital symptoms in individuals with a history of estrogen-dependent breast cancer: Clinical consensus. Obstet Gynecol. 2021;138(6):950–60.
61. Nappi RE, Kokot-Kierepa M. Women's voices in the menopause: Results from an international survey on vaginal atrophy. Maturitas. 2010;67(3):233–8.
62. Lester J et al. A self-report instrument that describes urogenital atrophy symptoms in breast cancer survivors. Western J Nursing Res. 2012;34(1):72–96.
63. Bygdeman M, Swahn ML. Replens versus dienoestrol cream in the symptomatic treatment of vaginal atrophy in postmenopausal women. Maturitas. 1996;23(3):259–63.
64. Seav SM et al. Management of sexual dysfunction in breast cancer survivors: A systematic review. Women's Mid-Life Health. 2015;1:9.
65. Hershman DL et al. Prevention of bone loss by zoledronic acid in premenopausal women undergoing adjuvant chemotherapy persist up to one year following discontinuing treatment. J Clin Endocrinol Metab. 2010;95(2):559–66.
66. Sverrisdóttir A et al. Bone mineral density among premenopausal women with early breast cancer in a randomized trial of adjuvant endocrine therapy. J Clin Oncol. 2004;22(18):3694–9.
67. Genant HK et al. Quantitative computed tomography of vertebral spongiosa: A sensitive method for detecting early bone loss after oophorectomy. Ann Intern Med. 1982;97(5):699–705.
68. Xu J et al. The recent progress of endocrine therapy-induced osteoporosis in estrogen-positive breast cancer therapy. Front Oncol. 2023;13.
69. Fogelman I et al. Bone mineral density in premenopausal women treated for node-positive early breast cancer with 2 years of goserelin or 6 months of cyclophosphamide, methotrexate and 5-fluorouracil (CMF). Osteoporos Int. 2003;14(12):1001–6.
70. Shapiro CL et al. Management of osteoporosis in survivors of adult cancers with nonmetastatic disease: ASCO clinical practice guideline. J Clin Oncol. 2019;37(31):2916–46.
71. Mustian KM et al. Exercise recommendations for cancer-related fatigue, cognitive impairment, sleep problems, depression, pain, anxiety, and physical dysfunction: A review. Oncol Hematol Rev. 2012;8(2):81.
72. Cramp F et al. The effects of resistance training on quality of life in cancer: A systematic literature review and meta-analysis. Support Care Cancer. 2010;18(11):1367–76.
73. Schmitz KH et al. American college of sports medicine roundtable on exercise guidelines for cancer survivors. Med Sci Sports Exerc. 2010;42(7):1409–26.

74. Eisen A et al. Use of adjuvant bisphosphonates and other bone-modifying agents in breast cancer: ASCO-OH (CCO) guideline update. J Clin Oncol. 2022;40(7):787–800.
75. Gralow JR et al. Phase III randomized trial of bisphosphonates as adjuvant therapy in breast cancer: S0307. J Natl Cancer Instit. 2020;112(7):698–707.
76. Wilson C et al. Adjuvant zoledronic acid reduces fractures in breast cancer patients; an AZURE (BIG 01/04) study. Eur J Cancer. 2018;94:70–8.
77. Hershman DL et al. Early discontinuation and non-adherence to adjuvant hormonal therapy are associated with increased mortality in women with breast cancer. Breast Cancer Res Treat. 2011;126(2):529.

Chapter 4

Pharmacological Management of Menopausal Symptoms in Breast Cancer Survivors

Mridula A. George, Ana Ferrigno Guajardo
and Maryam B. Lustberg

Introduction

With recent advances in screening, early detection, and treatment options, breast cancer survivors are living longer. However, these patients endure debilitating menopausal side effects that significantly impact their quality of life and treatment adherence, ultimately affecting disease outcomes.

Women with hormone receptor-(HR) positive breast cancer are prescribed adjuvant endocrine therapy for five to ten years to reduce the risk of recurrence and death. Postmenopausal women who have experienced a loss of ovarian function are treated with anti-estrogen oral agents such as aromatase inhibitors (AIs) or selective estrogen receptor modulators (SERMs) like tamoxifen. A significant proportion of premenopausal women diagnosed with HR-positive breast cancers undergo ovarian function suppression (OFS) through gonadotropin-releasing hormone (GnRH) agonists, in addition to oral endocrine therapies. Younger premenopausal women with biologically aggressive HR-negative tumors are treated with cytotoxic chemotherapy that can lead to chemotherapy-induced ovarian failure.

These menopausal symptoms are frequently cited as the reason for early therapy discontinuation and non-adherence (1–3). Early discontinuation of endocrine therapy has been associated with an increased risk of recurrence compared to patients who adhere to their treatments, both in premenopausal and postmenopausal women (4–6). A systematic review of 26 studies that evaluated patient adherence to hormonal therapy found that the rate of adherence declined by 25.5% from the first to the fifth year of treatment (3).

While physicians are aware of the benefits of adjuvant endocrine therapy, the menopausal side effects experienced by the patient are often under-appreciated. Proactively managing the complex symptoms of estrogen blockade in patients, while adequately treating the primary malignancy, is crucial. Monitoring and management of these symptoms will improve patient adherence and quality of life (7, 8).

DOI: 10.1201/9781032631028-4

Prevalence of Menopausal Symptoms in Survivors

The majority of breast cancer survivors face a myriad of menopausal side effects, which negatively impact their quality of life. Estrogen receptor modulation affects the overall well-being of patients by inducing menopausal side effects and long-term sequelae of hypoestrogenism. The constellation of side effects from anti-estrogen therapy range from hot flashes, mood disorders, vaginal dryness, alopecia, and decreased libido, to long-term issues such as cognitive dysfunction, sleep disturbances, and decreased bone health (9).

The severity and persistence of therapy-related side effects can impact adherence to the recommended adjuvant endocrine therapy (10). Without adequate support from clinicians, patients may resort to self-management strategies that can negatively affect adherence (11). Among patients with moderate to low social support, clinical support has been shown to reduce the risk of non-adherence (12). In addition to adherence, completion of the planned course of endocrine therapy (persistence) is essential to reduce the risk of disease recurrence. Both non-adherence and non-persistence are associated with high risk of mortality (6).

A small retrospective study evaluated the option of agent switching versus management of side effects while continuing therapy with the same agent. The study found that switching was associated with poor long-term adherence (13). Management strategies need to be individually tailored to the specific side effect experienced by the patient (Figure 4.1). Most of the intervention strategies revolve around the off-label use of medications approved for other indications. This chapter will focus on the management of some of the menopausal side effects experienced by breast cancer survivors.

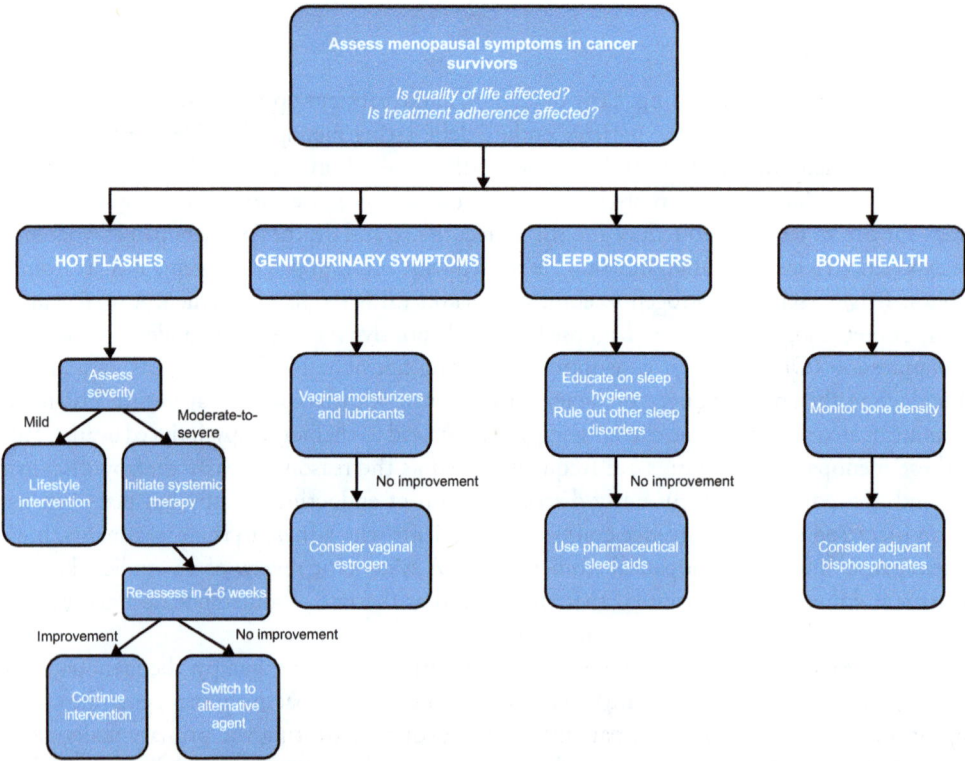

Figure 4.1 Management of menopausal side effects in breast cancer survivors.

Hot Flashes

Vasomotor symptoms (VMS), such as hot flashes, are the most common side effects of adjuvant therapies for breast cancer, which include ovarian function suppression, oral endocrine therapy (AI, SERD, or SERMs), and cytotoxic chemotherapy. Up to 95% of premenopausal women and 30% of postmenopausal women experience VMS (14–16). Furthermore, for postmenopausal women who have hot flashes pre-dating a breast cancer diagnosis, the initiation of cancer treatment can further exacerbate these symptoms (14). Estrogen withdrawal results in an increase of norepinephrine and serotonin release followed by instability of the hypothalamic thermoregulatory set point, which allows changes in the body temperature and in hot flash sensation.

VMS vary in duration and occur at any time of day. Hot flashes are a leading cause of treatment discontinuation in women taking adjuvant endocrine therapy (17). These symptoms result in nighttime awakenings, sleep disturbances, and impaired overall quality of life. Hence, women with moderate to severe VMS can benefit from pharmacologic therapies for management of symptom burden.

Hormonal Options

Hormonal therapy with estrogen is the first-line therapy for vasomotor symptoms in women without history of breast cancer. However, systemic hormonal replacement is contraindicated in women with hormone receptor-positive breast cancer given the increased risk of disease recurrence. Three independent randomized trials have evaluated the effects of estrogen and progesterone supplementation after a diagnosis of breast cancer: the Hormonal Replacement After Breast Cancer—Is it Safe? (HABITS), the Stockholm trial, and the Liberate study. The Stockholm trial was prematurely stopped in 2003 when HABITS reported increased disease recurrence (18), which was attributed to high progestogen exposure (18, 19). In contrast, the Liberate study evaluated tibolone, a synthetic steroid with weak estrogen, progestogen, and androgen activity, in breast cancer survivors. This study showed that tibolone relieved vasomotor symptoms and prevented bone loss, but at the cost of increased risk of breast cancer recurrence (20). Based on these three studies, hormone replacement therapy (HRT), alternatively known as menopausal hormone therapy (MHT), is contraindicated in breast cancer survivors with hormone-sensitive disease.

For hormone receptor-negative disease, the safety of HRT remains uncertain. Alternative pathways for estrogen and progestogen effects exist, including receptor conversion. A meta-analysis found ER and PR negative-to-positive conversion rates of 21.5% and 15.9%, respectively, in metastatic disease, while a prospective cohort found a hormone receptor negative-to-positive conversion rate of 13.9% after neoadjuvant chemotherapy in patients with residual disease (21). Furthermore, there is a theoretical concern of HRT stimulating healthy mammary epithelial cells expressing PR to produce RANKL, potentially promoting proliferation of HR-negative tumor cells via paracrine signaling (22). Given the aggressive nature of hormone receptor-negative disease and increased risk of second primary breast cancer, HRT is not routinely recommended, especially in younger patients, particularly in the first five years since diagnosis when recurrences are most likely to occur in hormone receptor-negative tumors (22). A recent meta-analysis of randomized clinical trials did not show a statistically significant increase in disease recurrence (HR 1.19, 95% CI 0.80–1.77, p = 0.390) in patients with hormone receptor-negative tumors treated with HRT (23). Hence, shared decision making can be used to discuss this as an option in certain patients with hormone receptor-negative tumors with high symptom burden.

An alternative to estrogen and progesterone replacement therapy is treatment with transdermal or subcutaneous testosterone, which has been shown to be effective in a small study (24).

However, due to limited data, testosterone implants are not commonly used. Caution is warranted because testosterone can be converted into estradiol by the enzyme aromatase in both, pre- and postmenopausal women. Hence, there is a theoretical risk for increased rate of disease recurrence with its use.

Non-Hormonal Options

Various non-hormonal alternatives have been studied to improve VMS in breast cancer survivors. A systematic review that compared at least two non-hormonal agents for hot flashes reduction revealed that hot flash reduction did not differ by tamoxifen or aromatase inhibitor use (25).

Serotonin-norepinephrine reuptake inhibitors (SNRI) and selective serotonin reuptake inhibitors (SSRI) have been shown to reduce VMS by regulating central norepinephrine activity in the brain, particularly the hypothalamus. They have been found to reduce the frequency and severity of hot flashes by 48–62% in comparison to placebo (26–29). Venlafaxine is the most well studied of the SNRI class, reducing symptoms by up to 62% as compared to placebo, clonidine, or gabapentin (30). SSRIs are not considered a first-line intervention for patients on tamoxifen, because they can reduce the bioavailability of tamoxifen via CYP2D6 inhibition. Concurrent potent CYP2D6-inhibitors such as paroxetine, bupropion, and fluoxetine result in significant reduction in circulating endoxifen levels (the active metabolite of tamoxifen) in some women. Moderate CYP2D6 inhibitors include duloxetine, sertraline, and citalopram. Venlafaxine is a weak inhibitor of CYP2D6 inhibitors. A pooled patient data analysis evaluating SNRIs and SSRIs for management of VMS revealed that patients had significant reduction of hot flashes with paroxetine and venlafaxine, and less effective results from fluoxetine and sertraline (31). For patients who are on SSRI/SNRIs that are potent inhibitors of CYP2D6 prior to initiating treatment with tamoxifen such as paroxetine and fluoxetine, it is recommended to switch to an SSRI with minimal CYP2D6 inhibition such as citalopram or venlafaxine to avoid compromising its therapeutic effect.

Antiepileptic agents such as gabapentin and pregabalin are also effective in controlling hot flashes. In patients who also suffer from neuropathic pain, this may be a reasonable consideration. A randomized double blinded study evaluated two dose levels of gabapentin (300 mg daily vs 900 mg daily) to determine the dose effectiveness for management of hot flashes (32). The study found that higher dose of gabapentin (900 mg/day divided into three doses) was more effective than gabapentin 300 mg daily for controlling hot flash frequency and severity (32). It is essential to ascertain the temporal pattern of VSM. Nocturnal hot flashes can increase the risk of insomnia, mood disorders, and fatigue (33). For nighttime VMS, gabapentin given one hour before sleep is associated with a reduction in nighttime hot flashes (34). If patients have daytime VMS, then an additional morning dose of gabapentin can be added (34). Of note, a multi-center open-label, randomized, cross-over trial compared four weeks of venlafaxine versus gabapentin to determine patient preference for management of hot flashes. The study showed that a larger proportion of patients preferred venlafaxine (68%) compared to gabapentin (32%) (35).

Several other pharmacologic options exist for management of VMS. Clonidine, a centrally acting α-adrenergic agonist, is effective for the management of hot flashes both as a transdermal patch and as an oral agent (36, 37). However, given the risk for hypotension in a patient population that may already have greater risk of bone fractures, other options are usually preferred. Oxybutynin at low doses (2.5–5 mg twice daily) has also been studied but its use is limited by anticholinergic side effects such as dry mouth, difficulty urinating, and abdominal pain (38).

Fezolinetant is an NK3R agonist that is FDA approved for decreasing frequency and intensity of hot flashes in menopausal women. However, it has not yet been studied in cancer patients, and there is a relatively small risk of elevated liver transaminases that are usually transient and without associated liver damage. Upcoming studies will evaluate its safety and efficacy in the breast cancer survivor population. An additional targeted therapy option is elinzanetant, a selective NK1–3 antagonist that is currently in trials for the management of VMS. The OASIS4 is an ongoing study which is evaluating the benefit of elinzanetant in patients with breast cancer experiencing vasomotor symptoms from endocrine therapy (NCT05587296).

Mood Disorders

A substantial proportion of patients with breast cancer are diagnosed with comorbid mood disorders, with an estimated 42% of patients experiencing anxiety (39) and 30% suffering from depression (40). Because psychiatric comorbidity has been associated with decreased quality of life (41), prompt identification of depression and anxiety is crucial in the treatment of breast cancer. Pharmacologic treatments that have shown to be effective in this population include SSRIs, SNRIs, tricyclic antidepressants (TCAs), and other agents, with selection of a specific agent often based on local availability, cost, side effect profile, and comorbidities. For instance, patients who experience bothersome hot flashes might particularly benefit from SSRIs or SNRIs while patients with co-existing neuropathic pain could be preferentially treated with SNRIs or tricyclic antidepressants, and those with concurrent nausea, sleep disturbances, and poor appetite could be managed with mirtazapine (42).

A systematic review demonstrated that approximately 23% of breast cancer survivors are prescribed antidepressants (43). Nonetheless, clinicians must exert caution when prescribing antidepressants given potential drug interactions specifically with tamoxifen. As discussed previously, paroxetine, fluoxetine, duloxetine, and bupropion inhibit cytochrome P450 2D6 (CYP2D6), which metabolizes tamoxifen to its primary active metabolite (endoxifen) (42). Hence, concurrent use of tamoxifen with potent CYP2D6 inhibitors could theoretically increase the risk of disease recurrence and disease-specific mortality even though this has not been consistently demonstrated in the literature (44, 45). Therefore, current guidelines recommend the use of antidepressants with moderate to low CYP2D6 inhibition properties such as citalopram, escitalopram, venlafaxine, desvenlafaxine, low-dose sertraline (<150 mg/day), and mirtazapine as first-line agents (42).

Randomized placebo-controlled studies that have evaluated the use of pharmacologic therapy for mood disorders in breast cancer patients specifically have found that fluoxetine (46), mianserin (47), and paroxetine (29) decrease depressive symptoms, while amitriptyline (48), bupropion (49), desipramine (50), and sertraline (51) have not been found to be superior to placebo. However, available data could be limited by limited statistical power, suboptimal instruments to quantify symptom burden, and/or insufficient follow-up. To date, no randomized placebo-controlled studies have explored the alleviation of anxiety in breast cancer patients as the main objective, but a trial found a statistically significant decrease in anxiety levels after amitriptyline use for treatment of neuropathic pain (48).

Sexual Health/Genitourinary Symptoms

Sexual health concerns are highly prevalent in patients diagnosed with breast cancer, with approximately 75% of patients experiencing some degree of sexual dysfunction after diagnosis (52). Two of the most common concerns pertaining to sexual health include dyspareunia secondary to vulvovaginal atrophy and hypoactive sexual desire. Left untreated, these conditions can have a negative impact on quality of life, strain interpersonal relationships, and decrease psychosocial well-being. However, both issues can be successfully addressed through proper assessment, counseling, and medical management.

Vulvovaginal Atrophy

A stepwise approach to treatment of vulvovaginal atrophy is recommended, reserving pharmacologic modalities to patients in whom other treatments have failed to provide adequate relief (53). Over-the-counter vaginal moisturizers and lubricants are considered first-line treatment options for all patients. These non-hormonal options are not able to reverse the atrophy from estrogen deprivation, but they have the potential to alleviate symptoms by increasing vaginal moisture.

Randomized clinical trials and prospective cohort studies have proven that both vaginal moisturizers and lubricants result in improvement of vaginal dryness and dyspareunia (54–56). In general, products without additives, an osmolality lower than 380 mOsm/kg, and a pH between 3.8–4.5 are recommended to reduce the probability of exacerbating mucosal irritation (57). The use of vaginal moisturizers with hyaluronic acid or coconut oil given three to five times a week can improve vulvovaginal health (53). However, vaginal lubricants do not help with long-term vaginal moisture. During sexual intercourse, water-based (KY Jelly) or silicone-based vaginal lubricants are used to reduce discomfort.

For patients who continue to have moderate to severe genitourinary symptoms despite a trial of vaginal moisturizers and lubricants, medicated alternatives can be pursued. Topical lidocaine has been shown to result in significant reductions in dyspareunia when used prior to penetrative sexual activity and can be offered as next-line treatment (58). An alternative to HRT approved for the treatment of severe vulvovaginal atrophy in otherwise healthy postmenopausal patients is ospemifene, a selective estrogen modulator. While definitive evidence proving its safety in patients with breast cancer is lacking, it has been shown not to increase breast cancer events in a cohort study including 1,728 patients, of whom 58 had a prior history of breast cancer (59). Nonetheless, current guidelines advise against its use in patients with a history of hormone-sensitive malignancy pending more robust safety data (60).

Vaginal estrogen therapy (VET) is considered relatively safe and can be offered to patients who have not benefited from an adequate trial of non-hormonal treatments. While it is unknown to what extent systemic absorption is associated with increased breast cancer recurrence risk, it is important for clinicians to be aware that the level of serum estrogen is directly associated with the potency of the active ingredient (conjugated equine estrogens > estradiol > estrone > estriol) and amount applied (with creams leading to greater systemic absorption compared to other modalities) (57, 61). A recent cohort study that included 49,237 patients with a history of breast cancer showed that use of topical estrogen therapy was not associated with higher breast cancer-specific mortality (aHR 0.77; 95%CI, 0.63–0.94) (62). However, another cohort study that included 8,461 patients indicated a higher recurrence risk (aRR, 95%CI 1.04–1.85) for patients treated with VET and concurrent treatment with aromatase inhibitors (63). Hence, patients in whom VET is being considered must be engaged in shared decision making after carefully weighing the expected risks and benefits associated with this therapy. A hormonal alternative to VET is intravaginal dehydroepiandrosterone (DHEA) ovules, which have been shown to reduce dyspareunia in otherwise healthy postmenopausal women (57). However, a randomized clinical trial in cancer survivors failed to demonstrate its superiority when compared to a vaginal moisturizer after 12 weeks of use (64). Another option is intravaginal testosterone, which has been proposed in particular for patients undergoing treatment with aromatase inhibitors in an effort to decrease systemic estrogen exposure, with available data from randomized trials showing improved dyspareunia and vaginal atrophy (65, 66). The long-term safety of these therapies remains to be elucidated.

Given the limited data on the efficacy of intravaginal treatment with energy-based devices such as CO_2 and radioablative lasers, alternative options should be encouraged, and such interventions should not be pursued outside clinical trials.

Hypoactive Sexual Desire

Decrease in sexual desire is reported by 50–70% of patients with breast cancer (67). Treatment of this condition largely focuses on psychosocial interventions and management of vulvovaginal symptoms. In particular, dyspareunia can lead to diminished sexual desire, arousal difficulties, and relationship problems. Therefore, it is crucial to address vulvovaginal atrophy in women who experience hypoactive sexual desire disorder.

Pharmacologic interventions that have been proven to be effective in otherwise healthy postmenopausal women, such as transdermal testosterone and bupropion, have yielded negative results when studied in patients with breast cancer (67, 68). Flibanserin, a 5-HT1A agonist, 5-HT2A antagonist, and weak partial D4 agonist, has emerged as a potential treatment strategy since it was associated with a statistically significant improvement in sexual desire in a small prospective trial of patients with breast cancer (69). Other options proposed by current guidelines include buspirone and bremelanotide (60), though no data on their efficacy and safety in this population is currently available.

Bone Health

Women achieve peak bone mass at age thirty. Breast cancer therapies can exacerbate bone loss in addition to underlying risk factors such as genetics, smoking, reduced physical activity, and chronic steroid use (70). Patients with breast cancer have been found to have higher incidence of fractures than the general population (71). Bone is a dynamic tissue that is regulated by osteoclasts and osteoblasts, which in turn are dependent on estrogen. Breast cancer treatments such as aromatase inhibitors, GnRH agonists, and chemotherapy affect bone health by modulating estrogen levels. A prospective study that evaluated the risk of osteopenia and osteoporosis found that breast cancer survivors had a 68% higher risk of osteopenia and osteoporosis compared to cancer-free women (HR = 1.68, 95% CI = 1.12–2.50) (72). Some of the risk factors for increased risk of decreased bone density in breast cancer survivors were age ≤ 50 years, estrogen receptor-positive tumors, and treatment with aromatase inhibitors alone or chemotherapy plus any hormone therapy (72).

In premenopausal women, tamoxifen causes bone loss about 1–2% per year (73). However in postmenopausal women, tamoxifen increases bone density by about 1–2% per year (73, 74). In contrast, aromatase inhibitors cause bone loss of 2–3% per year (75). The rate of bone loss is much higher in premenopausal women who are on ovarian function suppression (OFS) or have chemotherapy-induced menopause, at 7.7% (76) and 7% (77), respectively. The addition of aromatase inhibitors to GnRH agonists increases the rate of bone loss (11% per year) and increases the risk of bone fractures (78, 79). The Suppression of Ovarian Function Trial (SOFT) and Tamoxifen and Exemestane Trial (TEXT) studies evaluated the role of adjuvant OFS in premenopausal women and showed a higher number of fractures during adjuvant endocrine therapy with OFS plus AIs (7.7%) as compared with OFS plus tamoxifen (6.0%) or tamoxifen alone (5.3%) (80).

It is important to monitor bone density and to identify the risk factors for osteoporosis and bone fractures. Calcium and vitamin D supplementation are commonly recommended for breast cancer survivors. Treatment with bisphosphonates is recommended in the adjuvant setting for postmeno-pausal women and those on OFS to reduce risk of bone recurrence (81). A meta-analysis by Early Breast Cancer Clinical Trials Group (EBCCTG) evaluated individual patient data of 18,766 women derived from 26 randomized trials with adjuvant bisphosphonate in breast cancer (82). The study showed that the use of adjuvant bisphosphonate reduced bone recurrence and breast cancer mortality in all breast cancer subtypes (82). Among the different bisphosphonates that were evaluated in the study, a similar benefit was observed for clodronate, zoledronic acid, and ibandronate, whereas there was no apparent effect noted with pamidronate (82). Despite the benefit of bisphosphonates, they are not commonly used in postmenopausal women or premenopausal women on OFS (83).

Given the risk of osteonecrosis of jaw associated with bisphosphonates, dentistry evaluation is recommended before starting treatment with adjuvant bisphosphonates. Patients should be advised to inform their dentists about the use of bisphosphonates and to avoid invasive dental procedures.

Although there is disease-related benefit seen with adjuvant bisphosphonates, the use of RANKL inhibitors such as denosumab is not recommended as adjuvant therapy for breast cancer given conflicting results from prospective trials. D-CARE was a randomized phase III study comparing denosumab 120 mg every three to four weeks and placebo, and it showed no difference in bone-metastases-free survival (84). In contrast, the ABCSG-18 study which evaluated denosumab 60 mg every six months versus placebo in postmenopausal women who were on aromatase inhibitors showed an improvement in bone-metastases-free survival by 2.5% (88.9 vs. 86.4%; hazard ratio, 0.81) (85).

Sleep

It is estimated that 30–50% of patients with cancer experience sleep disorders, of which the etiology is often multifactorial and includes treatment-related side effects, comorbid psychiatric diagnosis, and biologic changes (86). In contrast, the Study of Women's Health across the Nation (SWAN) study showed that prevalence of sleep disorders in the premenopausal age group ranges from 16% to 42%; in perimenopausal women prevalence varies from 39% to 47%; in postmeno-pausal females, the prevalence ranges from 35% to 60% (87).

For patients in whom a sleep disorder is suspected, current guidelines recommend that clinicians assess for contributing factors for which targeted treatment could be initiated such as pain, emotional distress, fatigue unrelated to sleep (e.g., secondary to anemia, endocrine dysfunction, or cardiac disease), substance use disorder, and medication-related side effects. Furthermore, those patients with specific sleep disorders such as obstructive sleep apnea and restless leg syndrome should be offered targeted therapy. In patients who suffer from other sleep disturbances, non-pharmacologic treatment with sleep hygiene education, regular exercise, and psychosocial interventions should be offered as first-line treatment. For those patients with refractory symptoms and significant symptom burden, pharmacotherapy can be considered.

For patients with persistent insomnia despite conservative treatment, available therapies include short-acting benzodiazepines such as lorazepam that help with sleep initiation, longer-acting benzodiazepines such as temazepam that aid with sleep initiation and maintenance, non-benzodiazepine hypnotics like zolpidem, zaleplon, and eszopiclone that assist with sleep initiation and, depending on half-life, can also increase total sleep time, melatonin receptor agonists like ramelteon that mostly support sleep initiation, and sedating tricyclic antidepressants such as doxepin that decrease sleep latency (86, 88). Other options include other antidepressants such as trazodone or mirtazapine, first-generation antihistamines like diphenhydramine, antiepileptics like gabapentin, and atypical antipsychotics like quetiapine or olanzapine (86, 88). When selecting a specific agent, clinicians must carefully consider expected benefits and side effects. For example, mirtazapine might be a good choice in patients with insomnia and decreased appetite or nausea (89), while gabapentin could be a better choice in patients with concurrent neuropathic pain and nocturnal hot flashes.

In patients with refractory daytime sedation, available pharmacologic therapies include stimulants such as methylphenidate or dextroamphetamine; psychostimulants like modafinil and caffeine could be considered (89).

Hair Thinning

Hair loss or thinning is often an underreported effect of treatment with endocrine-based cancer therapies, but can affect up to 25% of patients taking aromatase inhibitors and tamoxifen (90). It often presents as diffuse alopecia over the fronto-parietal area of the scalp, with or without frontal hairline recession similar to female androgenetic alopecia (91). A meta-analysis that evaluated the incidence of alopecia across 35 clinical trials (>13,000 patients on endocrine therapy for breast cancer) revealed an overall incidence of alopecia of 4.4%, with the highest incidence in patients treated with tamoxifen (25.4%) (92).

The CHANCE study was a single-center, prospective, longitudinal cohort study of non-metastatic breast cancer patients treated with cytotoxic chemotherapies and/or endocrine therapies (93). Patient were assessed six months after chemotherapy completion or one year after the initiation of endocrine therapy (93). Grade 1 persistent scalp alopecia and eyebrow/lash loss were noted in 16% and 35% of the patients, respectively, with a negative impact in quality of life (93).

A single-arm study evaluated the effectiveness of topical minoxidil 5% in treating alopecia related to adjuvant endocrine therapy. Minoxidil improved alopecia in 82% of the patients (91). 5α-reductase inhibitors and spironolactone have not been well studied in breast cancer given the concern of its effect on the estrogen pathway. A pooled data analysis revealed that there was no significant change in level of estrogen when using 5α-reductase inhibitors or spironolactone (94). Further studies are needed to determine the safety and efficacy of spironolactone and 5α-reductase inhibitors (topical and oral) for the management of endocrine therapy-associated alopecia.

Conclusion

Menopausal symptoms are common in women who are undergoing treatment for breast cancer or have received chemotherapy for other malignancies. The specific symptoms experienced by patients differ based on the menopausal status prior to initiation of therapy, and the type of treatments used in the management of the cancer. It is important to assess menopausal symptoms in cancer survivors since they can negatively affect quality of life and increase non-adherence with medications prescribed to reduce the risk of recurrence. In addition to pharmacologic options, smoking cessation, weight loss, and regular physical activity are important in management of these symptoms. There is a need for more randomized studies to improve the QoL related to menopausal side effects. With newer non-hormonal agents such as fezolinetant and similar class of drugs in clinical development for VMS, it is important to determine their tolerability, efficacy, and safety for patients receiving adjuvant endocrine therapy. Additional efforts should be geared toward implementation of guidelines to assess and manage menopausal side effects in breast cancer survivors.

PATIENT CASE

A 45-year-old premenopausal woman recently completed adjuvant chemotherapy for HR+/HER2- negative T2N1 breast cancer. Following surgery, she was treated with docetaxel and cyclophosphamide adjuvant chemotherapy. After completion of chemotherapy, she was started on adjuvant endocrine therapy with ovarian function suppression and letrozole.

At the time of her first follow-up visit, she states that she is having a hard time with the side effects of cancer treatments. She has persistent neuropathy in her feet secondary to the chemotherapy. Since starting letrozole and ovarian function suppression, she is experiencing nocturnal hot flashes, which wake her up at night and cause daytime fatigue.

Given these symptoms, her oncologist discusses the benefit of adding gabapentin for the management of hot flashes. The oncologists explains that gabapentin could also help relieve symptoms caused by the chemotherapy-induced peripheral neuropathy, and the patient agrees to a bedtime trial of gabapentin.

At the next follow-up visit at four weeks, the patient reports significant improvement in hot flashes. She is also sleeping much better, since the hot flashes are not waking her up at night. She has noticed mild improvement in the neuropathy. Her oncologist also assesses for daytime somnolence or possible side effects of gabapentin, and they agree to monitor the symptoms and jointly decide to continue the medication.

References

1. Hershman DL et al. Psychosocial factors related to non-persistence with adjuvant endocrine therapy among women with breast cancer: The Breast Cancer Quality of Care Study (BQUAL). Breast Cancer Res Treat. 2016;157(1):133–43.
2. Kadakia KC et al. Patient-reported outcomes and early discontinuation in aromatase inhibitor-treated postmenopausal women with early stage breast cancer. Oncologist. 2016;21(5):539–46.
3. Yussof I et al. Factors influencing five-year adherence to adjuvant endocrine therapy in breast cancer patients: A systematic review. Breast. 2022;62:22–35.
4. Collin LJ et al. Early discontinuation of endocrine therapy and recurrence of breast cancer among premenopausal women. Clin Cancer Res. 2021;27(5):1421–28.
5. Ejlertsen B et al. Excess mortality in postmenopausal high-risk women who only receive adjuvant endocrine therapy for estrogen receptor positive breast cancer. Acta Oncol. 2014;53(2):174–85.
6. Hershman DL et al. Early discontinuation and non-adherence to adjuvant hormonal therapy are associated with increased mortality in women with breast cancer. Breast Cancer Res Treat. 2011;126(2):529–37.
7. Oberguggenberger A et al. Is the toxicity of adjuvant aromatase inhibitor therapy underestimated? Complementary information from Patient-Reported Outcomes (PROs). Breast Cancer Res Treat. 2011;128(2):553–61.
8. Smith KL et al. Association of treatment-emergent symptoms identified by patient-reported outcomes with adjuvant endocrine therapy discontinuation. NPJ Breast Cancer. 2022;8(1):53.
9. Goldberg C et al. Ovarian suppression: Early menopause, late effects. Curr Oncol Rep. 2024; 26(5):427–38.
10. Cahir C et al. Identifying the determinants of adjuvant hormonal therapy medication taking behavior in women with stages I-III breast cancer: A systematic review and meta-analysis. Patient Educ Couns. 2015;S0738–3991(15)00234-7.

11. Peddie N et al. The impact of medication side effects on adherence and persistence to hormone therapy in breast cancer survivors: A qualitative systematic review and thematic synthesis. Breast. 2021;58:147–59.
12. Kroenke CH et al. Personal and clinical social support and adherence to adjuvant endocrine therapy among hormone receptor-positive breast cancer patients in an integrated health care system. Breast Cancer Res Treat. 2018;170(3):623–31.
13. Kuhn EP et al. Management of adjuvant endocrine therapy (AET) side effects in patients with breast cancer: A single cancer center experience. J Clin Oncol. 2023;41(16_suppl):e12503.
14. Howell A et al. Results of the ATAC (Arimidex, Tamoxifen, Alone or in Combination) trial after completion of 5 years' adjuvant treatment for breast cancer. Lancet. 2005;365(9453):60–2.
15. Pagani O et al. Adjuvant exemestane with ovarian suppression in premenopausal breast cancer. N Engl J Med. 2014;371(2):107–18.
16. Pagani O et al. Adjuvant exemestane with ovarian suppression in premenopausal breast cancer: Long-term follow-up of the combined TEXT and SOFT trials. J Clin Oncol. 2023;41(7):1376–82.
17. Bell RJ et al. Understanding discontinuation of oral adjuvant endocrine therapy by women with hormone receptor-positive invasive breast cancer nearly 4 years from diagnosis. Menopause. 2013;20(1):15–21.
18. Holmberg L et al. Increased risk of recurrence after hormone replacement therapy in breast cancer survivors (vol 100, pg 475, 2008). J Nati Cancer Inst. 2008;100(9):685.
19. Fahlen M et al. Hormone replacement therapy after breast cancer: 10 year follow up of the Stockholm randomised trial. Eur J Cancer. 2013;49(1):52–9.
20. Kenemans P et al. Safety and efficacy of tibolone in breast-cancer patients with vasomotor symptoms: A double-blind, randomised, non-inferiority trial. Lancet Oncol. 2009;10(2):135–46.
21. Jin X et al. Prognostic value of receptor conversion after neoadjuvant chemotherapy in breast cancer patients: A prospective observational study. Oncotarget. 2015;6(11):9600–11.
22. van Barele M et al. Estrogens and progestogens in triple negative breast cancer: Do they harm? Cancer (Basel). 2021;13(11):2506.
23. Poggio F et al. Safety of systemic hormone replacement therapy in breast cancer survivors: A systematic review and meta-analysis. Breast Cancer Res Treat. 2022;191(2):269–75.
24. Glaser RL et al. Efficacy of subcutaneous testosterone on menopausal symptoms in breast cancer survivors. J Clin Oncol. 2014;32(26_suppl):109.
25. Johns C et al. Informing hot flash treatment decisions for breast cancer survivors: A systematic review of randomized trials comparing active interventions. Breast Cancer Res Treat. 2016;156(3):415–26.
26. Barton DL et al. Phase III, placebo-controlled trial of three doses of citalopram for the treatment of hot flashes: NCCTG trial N05C9. J Clin Oncol. 2010;28(20):3278–83.
27. Loprinzi CL et al. Venlafaxine in management of hot flashes in survivors of breast cancer: A randomised controlled trial. Lancet. 2000;356(9247):2059–63.
28. Loprinzi CL et al. Phase III evaluation of fluoxetine for treatment of hot flashes. J Clin Oncol. 2002;20(6):1578–83.
29. Roscoe JA et al. Effect of paroxetine hydrochloride (Paxil) on fatigue and depression in breast cancer patients receiving chemotherapy. Breast Cancer Res Treat. 2005;89(3):243–9.
30. Ramaswami R et al. Venlafaxine in management of hot flashes in women with breast cancer: A systematic review and meta-analysis. Breast Cancer Res Treat. 2015;152(2):231–7.
31. Loprinzi CL et al. Newer antidepressants and gabapentin for hot flashes: An individual patient pooled analysis. J Clin Oncol. 2009;27(17):2831–7.
32. Pandya KJ et al. Gabapentin for hot flashes in 420 women with breast cancer: A randomised double-blind placebo-controlled trial. Lancet. 2005;366(9488):818–24.
33. Joffe H et al. Independent contributions of nocturnal hot flashes and sleep disturbance to depression in estrogen-deprived women. J Clin Endocrinol Metab. 2016;101(10):3847–55.
34. Santen RJ et al. Managing menopausal symptoms and associated clinical issues in breast cancer survivors. J Clin Endocrinol Metab. 2017;102(10):3647–61.
35. Bordeleau L et al. Multicenter, randomized, cross-over clinical trial of venlafaxine versus gabapentin for the management of hot flashes in breast cancer survivors. J Clin Oncol. 2010;28(35):5147–52.

36. Goldberg RM et al. Transdermal clonidine for ameliorating tamoxifen-induced hot flashes. J Clin Oncol. 1994;12(1):155–8.
37. Pandya KJ et al. Oral clonidine in postmenopausal patients with breast cancer experiencing tamoxifen-induced hot flashes: A University of Rochester Cancer Center Community Clinical Oncology Program study. Ann Intern Med. 2000;132(10):788–93.
38. Leon-Ferre RA et al. Oxybutynin vs Placebo for hot flashes in women with or without breast cancer: A randomized, double-blind clinical trial (ACCRU SC-1603). JNCI Cancer Spectr. 2020;4(1):pkz088.
39. Hashemi SM et al. Prevalence of anxiety among breast cancer patients: A systematic review and meta-analysis. Breast Cancer. 2020;27(2):166–78.
40. Javan Biparva A et al. Global depression in breast cancer patients: Systematic review and meta-analysis. PLoS One. 2023;18(7):e0287372.
41. Hutter N et al. Are depression and anxiety determinants or indicators of quality of life in breast cancer patients? Psychol Health Med. 2013;18(4):412–19.
42. Li M et al. Management of depression in patients with cancer: A clinical practice guideline. J Oncol Pract. 2016;12(8):747–56.
43. Sanjida S et al. A systematic review and meta-analysis of prescribing practices of antidepressants in cancer patients. Psychooncology. 2016;25(9):1002–16.
44. Ahern TP et al. No increase in breast cancer recurrence with concurrent use of tamoxifen and some-inhibiting medications. Cancer Epidemiol Biomark Prev. 2009;18(9):2562–4.
45. Azoulay L et al. Concurrent use of tamoxifen with CYP2D6 inhibitors and the risk of breast cancer recurrence. Breast Cancer Res Treat. 2011;126(3):695–703.
46. Navari RM et al. Treatment of depressive symptoms in patients with early stage breast cancer undergoing adjuvant therapy. Breast Cancer Res Treat. 2008;112(1):197–201.
47. van Heeringen K, Zivkov M. Pharmacological treatment of depression in cancer patients: A placebo-controlled study of mianserin. Br J Psychiatry. 1996;169(4):440–3.
48. Eija K et al. Amitriptyline effectively relieves neuropathic pain following treatment of breast cancer. Pain. 1996;64(2):293–302.
49. Nunez GR et al. Bupropion for control of hot flashes in breast cancer survivors: A prospective, double-blind, randomized, crossover, pilot phase II trial. J Pain Symptom Manage. 2013;45(6):969–79.
50. Musselman DL et al. A double-blind, multicenter, parallel-group study of paroxetine, desipramine, or placebo in breast cancer patients (stages I, II, III, and IV) with major depression. J Clin Psychiatry. 2006;67(2):288–96.
51. Kimmick GG et al. Randomized, double-blind, placebo-controlled, crossover study of sertraline (Zoloft) for the treatment of hot flashes in women with early stage breast cancer taking tamoxifen. Breast J. 2006;12(2):114–22.
52. Jing LW et al. Incidence and severity of sexual dysfunction among women with breast cancer: A meta-analysis based on female sexual function index. Support Care Cancer. 2019;27(4):1171–80.
53. Carter J et al. Interventions to address sexual problems in people with cancer: American Society of Clinical Oncology clinical practice guideline adaptation of cancer care ontario guideline. J Clin Oncol. 2018;36(5):492–511.
54. Loprinzi CL et al. Phase III randomized double-blind study to evaluate the efficacy of a polycarbophil-based vaginal moisturizer in women with breast cancer. J Clin Oncol. 1997;15(3):969–73.
55. Lee YK et al. Vaginal PH-balanced gel for the control of atrophic vaginitis among breast cancer survivors. Obstet Gynecol. 2011;117(4):922–7.
56. Seav SM et al. Management of sexual dysfunction in breast cancer survivors: A systematic review. Women's Mid-Life Health. 2015;1:9.
57. Faubion SS et al. Management of genitourinary syndrome of menopause in women with or at high risk for breast cancer: Consensus recommendations from the North American Menopause Society and the International Society for the Study of Women's Sexual Health. Menopause. 2018;25(6):596–608.
58. Goetsch MF et al. A practical solution for dyspareunia in breast cancer survivors: A randomized controlled trial. J Clin Oncol. 2015;33(30):3394–+.
59. Cai B et al. No increase in incidence or risk of recurrence of breast cancer in ospemifene-treated patients with vulvovaginal atrophy (VVA). Maturitas. 2020;142:38–44.

60. Melisko ME, Narus JB. Sexual function in cancer survivors: Updates to the NCCN guidelines for survivorship. J Natl Compr Canc Netw. 2016;14(5_suppl):685–9.
61. Sussman TA et al. Managing genitourinary syndrome of menopause in breast cancer survivors receiving endocrine therapy. J Oncol Pract. 2019;15(7):363–70.
62. McVicker L et al. Vaginal estrogen therapy use and survival in females with breast cancer. JAMA Oncol. 2024;10(1):103–8.
63. Cold S et al. Systemic or vaginal hormone therapy after early breast cancer: A Danish observational cohort study. J Natl Cancer Inst. 2022;114(10):1347–54.
64. Barton DL et al. Evaluating the efficacy of vaginal dehydroepiandrosterone for vaginal symptoms in postmenopausal cancer survivors: NCCTG N10C1 (Alliance). Support Care Cancer. 2018;26(2):643–50.
65. Witherby S et al. Topical testosterone for breast cancer patients with vaginal atrophy related to aromatase inhibitors: A phase I/II study. Oncologist. 2011;16(4):424–31.
66. Melisko ME et al. Vaginal testosterone cream vs estradiol vaginal ring for vaginal dryness or decreased libido in women receiving aromatase inhibitors for early-stage breast cancer: A randomized clinical trial. JAMA Oncol. 2017;3(3):313–19.
67. Barton DL et al. Randomized controlled phase II evaluation of two dose levels of bupropion versus placebo for sexual desire in female cancer survivors: NRG-CC004. J Clin Oncol. 2022;40(4):324–34.
68. Barton DL et al. Randomized controlled trial to evaluate transdermal testosterone in female cancer survivors with decreased libido: North Central Cancer Treatment Group protocol N02C3. J Natl Cancer Inst. 2007;99(9):672–9.
69. Goldfarb SB et al. Effect of flibanserin on libido in women with breast cancer on adjuvant endocrine therapy. J Clin Oncol. 2023;41(16_suppl):12015. doi:10.1200/JCO.2023.41.16_suppl.12015.
70. Shapiro CL. Osteoporosis: A long-term and late-effect of breast cancer treatments. Cancers (Basel). 2020;12(11):3094.
71. Stumpf U et al. Incidence of fractures in young women with breast cancer—a retrospective cohort study. J Bone Oncol. 2019;18:100254.
72. Ramin C et al. Evaluation of osteopenia and osteoporosis in younger breast cancer survivors compared with cancer-free women: A prospective cohort study. Breast Cancer Res. 2018;20(1):134.
73. Powles TJ et al. Effect of tamoxifen on bone mineral density measured by dual-energy x-ray absorptiometry in healthy premenopausal and postmenopausal women. J Clin Oncol. 1996;14(1):78–84.
74. Love RR et al. Effect of tamoxifen on lumbar spine bone mineral density in postmenopausal women after 5 years. Arch Intern Med. 1994;154(22):2585–8.
75. Eastell R et al. Effect of an aromatase inhibitor on BMD and bone turnover markers: 2-year results of the Anastrozole, Tamoxifen, Alone or in Combination (ATAC) trial (18233230). J Bone Miner Res. 2006;21(8):1215–23.
76. Fogelman I et al. Bone mineral density in premenopausal women treated for node-positive early breast cancer with 2 years of goserelin or 6 months of cyclophosphamide, methotrexate and 5-fluorouracil (CMF). Osteoporos Int. 2003;14(12):1001–6.
77. Shapiro CL et al. Ovarian failure after adjuvant chemotherapy is associated with rapid bone loss in women with early-stage breast cancer. J Clin Oncol. 2001;19(14):3306–11.
78. Gnant MF et al. Zoledronic acid prevents cancer treatment-induced bone loss in premenopausal women receiving adjuvant endocrine therapy for hormone-responsive breast cancer: A report from the Austrian Breast and Colorectal Cancer Study Group. J Clin Oncol. 2007;25(7):820–8.
79. Bernhard J et al. Patient-reported outcomes with adjuvant exemestane versus tamoxifen in premenopausal women with early breast cancer undergoing ovarian suppression (TEXT and SOFT): A combined analysis of two phase 3 randomised trials. Lancet Oncol. 2015;16(7):848–58.
80. Francis PA et al. Tailoring adjuvant endocrine therapy for premenopausal breast cancer. N Engl J Med. 2018;379(2):122–37.
81. Dhesy-Thind S et al. Use of adjuvant bisphosphonates and other bone-modifying agents in breast cancer: A cancer care Ontario and American Society of Clinical Oncology clinical practice guideline. J Clin Oncol. 2017;35(18):2062–81.

82. Early Breast Cancer Trialists' Collaborative Group. Adjuvant bisphosphonate treatment in early breast cancer: Meta-analyses of individual patient data from randomised trials. Lancet. 2015; 386(10001):1353–61.

83. Balic M et al. St. Gallen/Vienna 2019: A brief summary of the consensus discussion on the optimal primary breast cancer treatment. Breast Care (Basel). 2019;14(2):103–10.

84. Coleman R et al. Adjuvant denosumab in early breast cancer (D-CARE): An international, multicentre, randomised, controlled, phase 3 trial. Lancet Oncol. 2020;21(1):60–72.

85. Gnant M et al. Adjuvant denosumab in postmenopausal patients with hormone receptor-positive breast cancer (ABCSG-18): Disease-free survival results from a randomised, double-blind, placebo-controlled, phase 3 trial. Lancet Oncol. 2019;20(3):339–51.

86. Denlinger CS et al. Survivorship: Sleep disorders, version 1.2014. J Natl Compr Canc Netw. 2014;12(5):630–42.

87. Kravitz HM, Joffe H. Sleep during the perimenopause: A SWAN story. Obstet Gynecol Clin North Am. 2011;38(3):567–86.

88. Levy M et al. Palliative care version 1.2016. J Nat Comp Cancer Network. 2016;14(1):82–113.

89. Kim SW et al. Effectiveness of mirtazapine for nausea and insomnia in cancer patients with depression. Psychiatry Clin Neurosci. 2008;62(1):75–83.

90. Gallicchio L et al. Aromatase inhibitor therapy and hair loss among breast cancer survivors. Breast Cancer Res Treat. 2013;142(2):435–43.

91. Freites-Martinez A et al. Endocrine therapy-induced alopecia in patients with breast cancer. JAMA Dermatol. 2018;154(6):670–5.

92. Saggar V et al. Alopecia with endocrine therapies in patients with cancer. Oncologist. 2013; 18(10):126–34.

93. Lacouture ME et al. The CHANCE study: A prospective, longitudinal study of chemotherapy and hormonal therapy induced hair changes and alopecia, skin aging and nail changes in women with non-metastatic breast cancer. J Clin Oncol. 2018;36(15_suppl):e12500. doi:10.1200/JCO.2018.36.15_ suppl.e12500.

94. Rozner RN et al. Safety of 5alpha-reductase inhibitors and spironolactone in breast cancer patients receiving endocrine therapies. Breast Cancer Res Treat. 2019;174(1):15–26.

Chapter 5

Pelvic Floor Problems after Cancer Treatment

Tim Hillard

Introduction

Pelvic floor problems can pose a considerable burden on quality of life in any woman, but in those who have already undergone treatment for cancer these may pose a significant additional burden and present unique challenges in how they should be managed. This chapter firstly considers whether the cancer itself or its treatment impact the likelihood of a woman developing new pelvic floor problems or the severity of pre-existing pelvic floor problems. If so, are there ways in which that impact could be mitigated, and what are the treatment options available to deal with these? Secondly, the chapter explores whether the standard treatments for pelvic floor disorders have to be adjusted or modified in any way because of the previous cancer diagnosis or as a result of its treatment.

This chapter concentrates on female pelvic cancers because they are the ones most likely to have an impact on pelvic floor function. However, it is recognised that other cancers can impact pelvic floor function either directly through surgery or indirectly as a consequence of the widespread impact of chemotherapy and radiotherapy on bladder, bowel, sexual and ovarian function. The impact of cancer and its treatment on sexual function and ovarian function are discussed in other chapters.

In 2020, there were almost 1.4 million new cases of gynaecologic malignancies diagnosed worldwide (cervical, endometrial, ovarian, vulval and vaginal) with cervical cancer being the third most common female malignancy (1). In addition, there were a further 865,630 colorectal cancers and 573,278 bladder cancers. The treatment for any of these cancers can potentially have an adverse impact on pelvic floor function. Although there are wide variations in health care around the world, advances in the diagnosis and treatment of gynaecological cancers mean that in many parts of the world the overall five-year survival rate is now over 70% (so maintenance of quality of life and social and economic activity are important considerations) (2).

Pelvic floor disorders (PFD), which embrace a wide range of symptoms affecting the bladder, bowel and vagina (Table 5.1), have become a major public health issue in developed countries. The associated symptoms can have a significant negative impact on a person's quality of life and ability

DOI: 10.1201/9781032631028-5

Table 5.1 Pelvic Floor Disorders and Typical Symptoms

Organ	Disorder	Typical Symptoms
Bladder	Abnormal storage Abnormal sensation Abnormal voiding	Urinary incontinence: stress, urge Urinary frequency, nocturia Enuresis Urgency, dysuria Absent sensation Painful bladder Straining to void, poor stream Incomplete emptying Retention Recurrent UTIs
Vagina	Pelvic organ prolapse Cystocele Rectocele/enterocele Uterine prolapse Vault prolapse Vaginal stenosis Vaginal atrophy	Pelvic pressure Introital bulging Pelvic, low back pain Voiding difficulty Constipation Dyspareunia Apareunia Vaginal dryness, post-coital bleeding
Bowel	Abnormal storage Evacuatory disorders	Faecal urgency, incontinence Faecal soiling Constipation Incomplete evacuation

to function normally, which in turn can result in social isolation, relationship difficulties, potential loss of income and mental health problems. Given the impact these symptoms may have on top of the psychological burden of a diagnosis of cancer and any other effects of their treatment, these women deserve particular attention. Managing pelvic floor problems may well be outside the professional capabilities of the oncologists, nurses or surgeons looking after these women, but every effort should be made to make the necessary enquiries about these symptoms and engage with appropriate colleagues in urogynaecology, urology, colorectal and sexual health for their help and support.

Prevalence

Determining the prevalence of PFD in gynaecological cancer survivors (GCS) depends firstly on their prevalence before cancer treatment and secondly on any change in the prevalence after treatment. The overall prevalence of PFD in healthy, nonpregnant women is reported to be up to 25% (3) with a 31.6% prevalence of one or more PFDs in women aged 50–59. However, the prevalence of pelvic floor symptoms such as urinary incontinence amongst gynaecological cancer survivors appears to be higher than in the general population (4). Almost two thirds of women diagnosed with a gynaecologic malignancy reported experiencing symptoms of urinary incontinence (UI), prolapse or both before cancer treatment and around one fifth rated their symptoms as moderately to severely bothersome (5). Since it is the most common gynaecological cancer in developed countries, much of the data relate to endometrial cancer, and it is quite possible that the higher prevalence of pelvic floor disorders seen in these patients is associated with a commonality of risk factors such as obesity, age and comorbidities like diabetes and hypertension (4–6).

There are relatively few good-quality studies addressing the prevalence of pelvic floor symptoms amongst GCS, and interpretation of the data that are available is hampered by a wide range of differences in reporting, assessment of PFD, the populations and the cancers studied and a lack of comparative data with healthy controls. In a systematic review of 31 articles, Ramaseshan et al. (7) identified the prevalence of major pelvic floor symptoms before and after cancer treatment in survivors of the major gynaecological malignancies. There appeared to be an increase in many pelvic floor symptoms after cancer treatment (Table 5.2). The prevalence of each symptom varied dependent on the type of cancer, which in turn probably reflected the treatment modalities employed. In women with cervical cancer, they noted a 4–76% post-treatment prevalence of stress urinary incontinence, a 4–59% post-treatment prevalence of urge incontinence, and a 2–34% prevalence of faecal incontinence. Cervical cancer treatment also caused urinary retention 0.4–39% and dyspareunia 7–39%. In addition to an increased prevalence, it is important to recognise that pelvic floor dysfunction after cancer treatment is one of the principal causes of a reduced quality of life for many women (8).

In one of the few detailed observational studies of gynaecological cancer survivors, Neron et al. (9) reported that symptoms of faecal and urge incontinence and prolapse were significantly worse than in the general population (Figure 5.1) and that overall survivors of gynecological cancer experienced significantly more pelvic floor symptoms and an associated reduction in quality of life. Significantly higher rates of stress urinary incontinence (SUI), urge urinary incontinence (UUI), nocturia and urgency were also reported in survivors of endometrial and cervical cancer in comparison with the prevalence in women without cancer (10). Rutledge et al. (11) found that 67% of gynaecologic cancer survivors who were treatment-free for more than a year reported moderate to severe urinary incontinence. Faecal incontinence and sexual dysfunction were also significant problems. Manchana et al. (12) reported that up to two thirds of cervical cancer survivors after

Table 5.2 Prevalence (%) of Pelvic Floor Disorders in Patients with Gynaecologic Malignancy before and after Treatment.

Type of cancer	No. of patients	Treatment status	SUI (%)	UUI (%)	UR (%)	FI (%)	POP (%)
Cervical	2,875	Before	24–29	8–18	NR	6	16
		After	4–76	3–59	0.4–39	2–34	NR
Uterine	2,977	Before	29–36	15–25	NR	3	7
		After	69–84	67–80	NR	11–24	44
Ovarian	375	Before	32–42	15–39	NR	4	17
		After	NR	NR	NR	7	NR
Vulvar	604	Before	44	22	NR	0	NR
		After	NR	NR	NR	1–20	1–16

Source: Adapted from Ramaseshan AS et al. (2018)

Note: SUI—stress urinary incontinence
    UUI—urgency urinary incontinence
    UR—urinary retention
    FI—fecal incontinence
    POP—pelvic organ prolapse
    NR—not reported

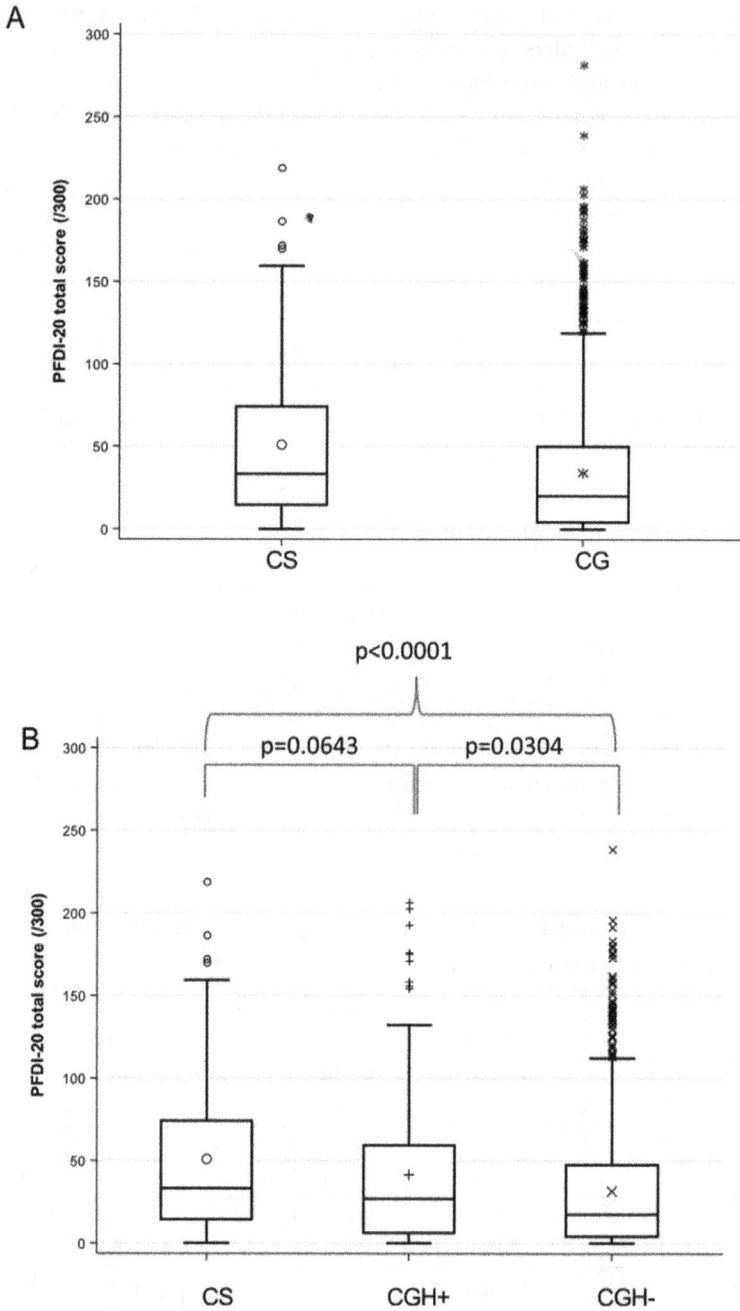

Figure 5.1 Boxplot comparing Pelvic Floor Distress Index-20 global score of A) cancer survivors (CS) to control group (CG) and B) cancer survivors (CS) to women who underwent benign hysterectomy (CGH+) and women with no history of cancer or hysterectomy (CGH–). Global scores range from 0–300; the higher scores represent more symptoms and associated discomfort.

(Reproduced from Neron et al. (9) under a Creative Commons Attribution 4.0 International License.)

radical hysterectomy had urodynamic abnormalities. Half of them had voiding dysfunction and one third had storage dysfunction. Some researchers noted that urinary incontinence rates tended to be highest in the early post-operative period. Ceccaroni et al. found a urinary incontinence rate of 55% at 1 month after surgery (13), while Naik et al. found urinary incontinence rates of 48% and 17% respectively at 1.5 months and after 12 months after surgery (14). There is little published data on longer-term outcomes.

Pelvic organ prolapse (POP) is a common postoperative complication in GCS, usually presenting as prolapse of the anterior and posterior vaginal walls, vaginal vault, uterus, and bladder (15), and the reported incidence after hysterectomy may be as high as 39% (16). Faecal incontinence (FI) is a common and distressing symptom that occurs in up to 43% of GCS that may develop several years after the completion of cancer treatment (17).

Overall, the data seem to indicate that pelvic floor symptoms are more prevalent in the gynaecological cancer population, quite possibly due to overlapping risk factors. There may be an additional increased incidence after treatment which is likely to vary depending on the nature of treatment, which in turn will depend on the original site of the cancer. Assessing the prevalence of pelvic floor problems in cancer survivors may be further complicated because these symptoms are often more tolerated, if not totally neglected, by many cancer survivors (18). Interestingly these findings may be specific to gynaecological cancers since amongst breast cancer survivors the prevalence of pelvic floor disorders was actually lower than controls in one study (19), although the rates of surgical intervention were increased for some conditions. However, other studies have found differing results (20).

Colorectal cancer can also be associated with PFD, and the highest proportions are seen in patients receiving primary radiotherapy (21).

Impact of Treatment

Cancer treatment of any sort can impact pelvic floor function either directly during surgical intervention or radiotherapy or indirectly via chemotherapy. If the ovaries are removed or rendered inactive by the treatment this will lead to loss of oestrogen which in turn can result in weakening of pelvic floor structures and the symptoms of genito-urinary syndrome of menopause. This is discussed further in Chapters 4 and 6. This next section explores the impact different cancer treatment modalities may have on pelvic floor function.

Surgery

Cancer surgery, by necessity, is often fairly radical, and its impact on the pelvic floor will likely depend on the extent of any surgery. The treatment for many pelvic cancers involves organ removal such as a hysterectomy, often combined with a bilateral salpingo-oophorectomy. Hysterectomy itself can cause weakening and displacement of the some of the supporting fascia and ligaments of the pelvis, increasing the possibility of subsequent prolapse (22).

Bladder function may be impacted by denervation during surgery leading to altered sensation to void which may manifest as urinary frequency and/or urinary urgency with incontinence. It may also impact voiding function; voiding difficulties are common after radical pelvic surgery and careful postoperative bladder management is necessary to recognise and manage this. Bowel function can also be disrupted because pelvic denervation may result in reduced sensation of fullness and increased evacuatory difficulties. Faecal urgency and incontinence were significantly worse in cancer survivors than the general population (9). If radical surgery involves resection of part or all of the bladder, rectum or sigmoid colon, that is likely to involve the creation of a temporary or permanent urinary diversion into a pouch or a stoma, which clearly has a major impact on subsequent pelvic floor function.

Any surgery that results in removal of the upper part of the vagina, either by design or due to surgical difficulties, may compromise vaginal length and function. This potentially has an impact on sexual function, which is explored elsewhere (Chapter 6) but may also compromise future pelvic floor treatment if needed.

Surgical complications are a recognised part of any pelvic surgical procedure, and with potentially invasive cancer, the risks are inevitably higher. Complications such as urinary tract infections, bladder, ureteric or bowel damage, fistula formation or excessive scarring from a haematoma are all real possibilities that could have a potential impact on future pelvic floor function.

After surgery for gynaecological cancer, women had significantly more pelvic floor symptoms compared with the general population, including those who had undergone a hysterectomy for benign indications. However, the impact of hysterectomy on PFD is still debated. Whilst hysterectomy did have an impact on pelvic floor symptoms and quality of life, this impact does not appear to be as significant as the cancer itself (Figure 5.1) (9). Assessing the true impact of hysterectomy on pelvic floor function can be confounded by whether it is carried out in isolation or combined with adjuvant treatment such as radiotherapy. In addition, advances in surgical technique, such as robotic surgery, may lead to fewer complications, but few data are currently available.

Radical hysterectomy is considered one of the main causes of rectal dysfunction in patients. The pudendal nerve that innervates the anal sphincter, as well as the sympathetic and para-sympathetic nerves, may be damaged during the operation, which affects the innervation of the ano-rectal nerve and causes symptoms such as anal incontinence (23).

Radiotherapy

Radiotherapy, either alone or in combination with chemotherapy and/or surgery, is commonly used in the treatment of lower abdominal and pelvic cancers. By its very nature radiotherapy destroys not only the cancer cells in the field of treatment but also healthy cells in the surrounding area. Recent advances in radiotherapy, such as intensity-modulated radiotherapy (IMRT), conformal radiotherapy (CRT), image guided brachytherapy and high-energy linear accelerators allow more targeted radiation to the tumour itself and try to limit the collateral damage to healthy tissues, but there are still inevitably some unwanted effects (24, 25). The extent of any healthy tissue damage will depend on multiple factors including the radiation dose used, the interval between treatments and the radiosensitivity of the surrounding tissues. Some of these factors can be modified to protect healthy tissue by the use of hyper-fractionation when a high total dose of radiation is given over a larger number of small doses per fraction. Because normal tissues can repair radiation damage more effectively than cancer cells, the smaller doses allow better healing.

Complications of radiotherapy are generally considered to be either acute (within 90 days) or late (chronic), which can occur many years later. Acute radiation damage predominantly affects rapidly proliferating cells such as epithelial surfaces of the skin or gastrointestinal tract. The radiation damages the stem cells so there is inadequate cell turnover and a loss of the protective barrier. The symptoms usually resolve over a few weeks, but if the damage fails to heal, then symptoms may persist into the chronic phase (26). Late complications, on the other hand, tend to occur in tissues with slower turnover such as muscle, subcutaneous tissue and the wall of the intestine. Here, radiation leads to atrophy and necrosis with vascular damage and fibrosis. Carcinogenesis may also develop. In addition, co-existing comorbidities, such as raised BMI, anaemia, diabetes or circulatory disorders, may increase the risk of chronic radiation injury.

Although radiation complications can affect all the pelvic structures to a varying degree, for clarity they are split into individual components.

Bladder Effects

Ulceration of the bladder after radium treatment for uterine cancer was first described almost 100 years ago (27). The bladder and ureters are the most susceptible to radiation complications, which include haemorrhagic cystitis, urethral and ureteral strictures, urinary fistulae and the development of secondary primary malignancies (24). Bladder fibrosis and necrosis can also occur, which may lead to chronic renal dysfunction. The most common adverse events are radiation cystitis, ureteral stenosis and vesicovaginal fistula (24).

Genitourinary complications of radiotherapy can be graded 1–5 according to the Radiation Therapy Oncology Group (RTOG)/European Organisation for Research and Treatment of Cancer (EORTC) (Cox) (28) and are listed in Table 5.3. Other grading systems such as the National Cancer Institute Common Terminology Criteria for Adverse Events (NCI CTCAE) can also be used (29). Most complications are mild (grade 1–2), but more severe complications can occur particularly after cervical or bladder cancer treatment.

Several large institutional series reported grade 1 and 2 late bladder complications in 28% to 45% of patients after definitive RT for cervical cancer, whereas severe bladder dysfunction was relatively uncommon (30). Parkin et al. noted a 26% incidence of severe urgency, frequency and incontinence after RT for cervical cancer. Urodynamics performed before and after treatment

Table 5.3   Bladder Complications

	ACUTE	LATE
GRADE 1	Frequency of urination or nocturia twice pre-treatment habit/dysuria, urgency not requiring medication	Any slight epithelial atrophy, microscopic haematuria and mild telangiectasia
GRADE 2	Frequency of urination or nocturia that is less frequent than every hour. Dysuria, urgency, bladder spasm requiring local anaesthetic (e.g., Pyridium)	Any moderate frequency, generalised telangiectasia, intermittent macroscopic haematuria and intermittent incontinence
GRADE 3	Frequency with urgency and nocturia hourly or more frequently/dysuria, pelvis pain or bladder spasm requiring regular, frequent narcotic/gross haematuria with/without clot passage	Any severe frequency and urgency, severe telangiectasia, persistent incontinence, reduced bladder capacity (<150 ml) and frequent haematuria
GRADE 4	Haematuria requiring transfusion/acute bladder obstruction not secondary to clot passage, ulceration or necrosis	Any necrosis, fistula and haemorrhagic cystitis, bladder capacity (<100 ml), refractory incontinence requiring catheter or surgical intervention
GRADE 5	Death	Death

Source: Cox, JD, et. al. (1995)

revealed no differences in postvoid residual or maximum flow rate, although there were decreases in maximum bladder capacity and bladder compliance (31). In a series of 141 patients with cervical cancer who received MR-guided brachytherapy, Georg et al. (32) noted a dose-response relationship with side effects. The rate of grade 1 and 2 late complications was 16%, and the rate of grade 3 and 4 late complications requiring cystectomy was 1.4%.

Others have reported the incidence of mild late complications (RTOG Grade 1–2) after radiation for cervical cancer at just under 10% and after radiotherapy for endometrial cancer between 11–17% (24, 25, 30, 33). The incidence of more severe late complications (RTOG grade 3–4) is 1.3–14.5% after cervical cancer and most commonly include ureteral stricture and haemorrhagic cystitis. Serious bladder complications up to five years after treatment for endometrial cancer are rare probably due to the use of a single radiation modality (external beam radiotherapy [EBRT] or brachytherapy) and a relatively moderate dose. In patients with medically inoperable endometrial cancer who receive HDR brachytherapy, the reported major complications rate is 6% (30).

Clinical Presentation

Acute radiation cystitis usually presents as increased urinary frequency and urgency with dysuria. It is common after radiotherapy occurring in around 5–10% of people undergoing pelvic irradiation (34). It is usually self-limiting (up to three months), but damage to the urothelium can lead to inflammatory changes in the deeper tissues (35). The typical cystoscopy appearances are hyperaemia and oedema with signs of urothelial inflammation or an atrophic mucosa with telangiectasia (Figure 5.2a and 5.2b).

Chronic radiation cystitis, or chronic haemorrhagic cystitis, is relatively uncommon but is a progressive and irreversible condition that can occur up to 20 years after irradiation (24). It is characterised by haematuria which can vary from mild haematuria, through to significant haematuria with clot formation causing urinary retention, all the way through to life-threatening haemorrhage. It is also associated with other common lower urinary tract symptoms such as frequency, urgency, nocturia, dysuria and urinary incontinence. In addition, there may be suprapubic pain and generalised fatigue. These symptoms can have a big impact on a patient's quality of life and in

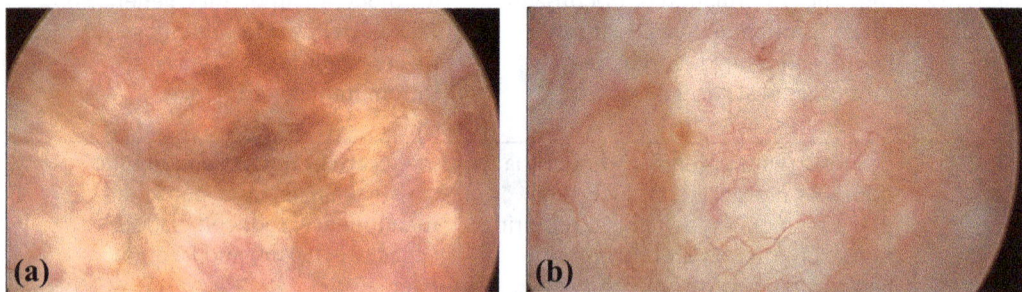

Figure 5.2 Typical cystoscopic findings of late radiation damage.
a) erythema, oedema, bleeding ulcers and fibrosis leading to reduced bladder capacity
b) atrophic mucosa and telangiectatic blood vessels

(Reproduced with permission from D'Ancona et al. (25) under a Creative Commons Attribution 3.0 License.)

rare situations be life-threatening (36). Chronic radiation cystitis is also very difficult to treat (see the following), which adds to the burden of the condition which can be overwhelming at times and result in frequent attendance at emergency clinics (37). Because these symptoms are quite non-specific, other causes of haematuria should be excluded with appropriate investigations including full vaginal examination to exclude a fistula, imaging of the upper and lower urinary tract and cystoscopy with biopsy. With the latter there is an increased risk of bladder wall perforation due to the relatively poor healing of the tissues. Urodynamic studies may also be useful to assess cystometric capacity, detrusor compliance, sphincter compliance and urethral closure pressures.

In radiation cystitis the tissues become hypovascular, hypocellular and hypoxic (so-called "three-H tissue") (24, 38). This is thought to be secondary to obliterative endarteritis (39), and the subsequent hypoxia results in mucosal necrosis causing haematuria. Further necrosis of the detrusor muscle increases the possibility of fistula formation. Ischemia of the bladder wall results in progressive fibrosis with resulting reduced bladder capacity and urinary incontinence. Telangiectasia can also develop and the fragile dilated vessels can lead to haematuria and pain.

Other Urinary Tract Effects

Vesico-Vaginal Fistula

Although uncommon, these fistulas can be devasting and because of the poor quality of the surrounding tissues they can be very difficult to treat. They occur in 1–10% of people undergoing pelvic radiotherapy and can occur many years after the initial treatment (24). The fistulas are often multiple or large and most commonly occur in the trigone. Entero-vesical fistulas can also develop, most commonly with the colon. Recto-vesical fistulas are more common after irradiation for prostate cancer. The diagnosis is made on examination with a high index of suspicion, followed by appropriate imaging such as cystography, CT scans (Figure 5.3a, 5.3b) (40) and cystoscopy with dye such as methylene blue.

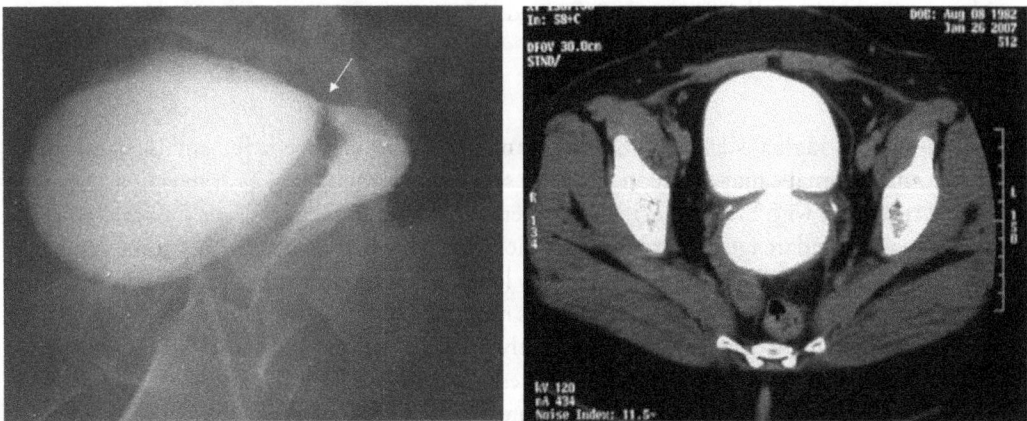

Figure 5.3   Imaging of vesico-vaginal fistula.
a) Cystography (lateral image). The *arrow* demonstrates the vesicovaginal fistula tract.
b) CT scan of vesicovaginal fistula. After the intravenous administration of the contrast agent, there is high-density material in both the bladder and the vagina, consistent with a VVF.

(Reproduced from Stamatokos M et al. (40) with permission.)

Ureteral Stricture

Ureteral stricture is rare but may be associated with cervical cancer with a reported incidence of 3.3% within 25 years after treatment with an average latency of almost 17 years (41). The typical site is 4–6 cm proximal to the ureteric orifice and caused by progressive fibrosis. These are often asymptomatic and detected by chance and may be accompanied by hydronephrosis and vesico-ureteric reflux. Given that many women undergoing treatment for cervical cancer are young, the long latent period is something that needs to be borne in mind when women present with hypertension or impaired renal function in later life.

Urethral Strictures

This is very uncommon in women and usually occurs in men after treatment for prostate cancer. However, it should be considered in women presenting with symptoms of voiding dysfunction who have a history of pelvic irradiation.

Bowel Effects

As with the bladder effects, radiation injury to the bowel can be divided into an acute and a chronic phase. An acute injury occurs within six weeks of the radiation treatment and is associated with faecal urgency, diarrhoea, faecal incontinence and rectal bleeding. There may also be decreased mucus production and submucosal oedema due to the effects of the radiation on the mucosa of the colon and rectum. The symptoms usually settle fairly quickly once the radiation treatment has finished. Chronic radiation proctitis is common, occurring in up to 75% of patients receiving pelvic radiation therapy (30). The symptoms are similar to those experienced with acute injury although bleeding is more usual, and again, they can develop many years after the initial radiation. Colonoscopy findings may include evidence of inflammation, ulcerations and strictures. The pathophysiology is the same as the bladder with ischaemia and fibrosis, and care should be taken with any biopsy because of the increased risk of perforation.

Vaginal Stenosis

Radiation-induced vaginal stenosis (VS) is a common side effect of pelvic RT and is characterised as an abnormal vaginal canal obstruction due to scar tissue formation (42). It mostly occurs after combined treatment with brachytherapy and external beam radiotherapy (EBRT). Brachytherapy tends to cause tissue damage throughout the whole vagina, whereas with ERBT some areas may be affected more than others. Radiation causes local inflammation with vaginal epithelial and connective tissue damage leading to fibrosis. This results in a dry, less elastic and shortened vagina. Pelvic irradiation can also cause fibrosis of the pelvic floor ligaments and muscles, which may also lead to shortening or narrowing of the vagina. These changes will have an effect on sexual function (discussed in Chapter 6) and may also be associated with pelvic pain and urinary incontinence.

Secondary Radiation-Induced Cancers

These are rare and can occur many years later. They are different histologically from the original tumour and are a result of carcinogenic mutations caused by the initial radiation. Secondary primary bladder cancers have also been reported (24).

Chemotherapy

Bladder symptoms are a common side effect of chemotherapy. Many of the commonly used agents such as cyclophosphamide, busulfan, and cabazitaxel are excreted in the urine as substances that can irritate the bladder mucosa. Typical symptoms include urinary frequency and urgency, and intense pain sometimes associated with haematuria. Some agents can also cause discolouration of the urine for 24 hours or so after treatment. By their very nature, chemotherapy agents are given systemically so chemotherapy for any cancer in the body may have an impact on the bladder in particular either during treatment or many years later, even after childhood cancer (43). Lower urinary tract symptoms, particularly nocturia, are common with certain chemotherapy agents, which may be secondary to chemotherapy-induced peripheral neuropathy (44).

Specific Considerations

Many of the effects of pelvic cancer treatment on pelvic floor symptoms are generic but there are some additional considerations depending on the type of cancer being treated.

Cervical Cancer

Cervical cancer often requires radical surgery and/or radiotherapy. As discussed earlier, both have their own complications associated with them, but the combination of surgery and radiotherapy together seems to be associated with a higher rate of severe urological complications (24). In a comparative study between different modalities using the Urinary Distress Inventory (UDI), Hazelwinkel et al. (45) reported stress urinary incontinence rates up to 11 years after treatment of 53% for radiotherapy alone, 60% after surgery and 76% after combined treatment. The same study found urge urinary incontinence rates were similar in the combined group (58%) compared with radiotherapy alone (57%) but lower in the surgery group (45%).

As might be expected, nerve-sparing radical hysterectomy (NSRH) seems to be associated with lower rates of subsequent bladder problems than radical hysterectomy (RH). Ceccaroni et al. (46) reported a 55% rate of UI after RH compared with just 8% after NSRH. In the same study the incidence of significant postvoid residuals (>100mls) was 39% in the RH group and 8% after NSRH. What impact radical robotic hysterectomy has on subsequent bladder dysfunction has not yet been fully assessed, but given the apparent benefits of NSRH it can be expected to provide a similar level of benefit. Urological complications in non-cancer patients seem similar between laparoscopic and robotic hysterectomy (47).

The risk of vaginal stenosis after radiotherapy seems to be related to the volume of vagina treated. In the EMBRACE study for cervical cancer, the 24-month estimate for symptomatic vaginal stenosis was 21%, with the extent of the tumour into the vagina being a considerable risk factor (48). In the first three years after pelvic radiotherapy for endometrial, cervical and anorectal cancer, the estimated rates of vaginal stenosis are 50%, 60% and 80% respectively (42). It occurs most commonly after combined treatment with brachytherapy and external beam radiotherapy.

Endometrial Cancer

Endometrial cancer tends to present earlier, and the surgical treatment may be less radical, so the potential impact of the cancer surgery *per se* over and above a benign hysterectomy is probably limited. If more radical surgery is required, the use of nerve sparing techniques, either laparoscopically or robotically, are likely to minimise the impact on pelvic floor function.

As with cervical cancer, the combination of different treatment modalities appears to have a more negative impact on pelvic floor function. In the PORTEC-1 Trial (Postoperative Radiation Therapy in Endometrial Carcinoma), urinary incontinence (based on patient-reported pad usage) was reported by 15% of women who underwent surgery but 43% of women who underwent surgery plus external beam radiation therapy (EBRT) (49). In the PORTEC-2 Trial which compared vaginal brachytherapy for local disease with EBRT, the urinary incontinence rates were similar between the two groups at seven years (41% and 44%). However, the faecal urgency and faecal incontinence rates were lower for the brachytherapy group (32% and 15% respectively) than for the ERBT group (55% and 24%) (50).

Only one study has evaluated prolapse in women after hysterectomy for endometrial cancer (51). In a cross-sectional study of 25 women, pelvic organ prolapse was identified in 44% six months after surgery.

Characteristically women with endometrial cancer might be expected to be over 60 and have a high BMI and multiple co-morbidities, all of which are risk factors for pelvic floor disorders. It is thus perhaps not surprising there appears to be a high incidence of pelvic floor disorders in this group, and many of these women may require pelvic floor intervention of some sort irrespective of their cancer diagnosis.

Ovarian Cancer

There are very few data regarding pelvic floor disorders in women who have had ovarian cancer quite probably because of the relatively late diagnosis in many cases and relatively poor five-year survival. Cross-sectional data suggests a baseline prevalence of stress urinary incontinence of 32%–42%, urge urinary incontinence 15%–39% and prolapse 17% (7).

Vulval Cancer

Radical vulvectomy by its very nature has the potential to have an impact on bladder, bowel and sexual function. Again, data are limited to cross-sectional and retrospective studies. The type of vulvectomy and the use of adjuvant therapy may make a difference (7). One study found a 6% incidence of stress urinary incontinence after a radical vulvectomy, 19% after a three-incision radical vulvectomy and 20% in those who underwent an en bloc radical vulvectomy (52). In a case control study of 40 women who had either surgery alone or surgery with chemoradiotherapy, 25% of women who underwent surgery with partial urethral resection reported urinary incontinence (using the standardised International Incontinence Questionnaire) and 25% reported spraying (53). In those who did not have a partial urethral resection only 5% reported urinary incontinence and 10% spraying. In the group who had surgery and chemoradiotherapy 29% reported urinary incontinence and 14% spraying. Anal incontinence is also reported in some patients (54).

Colorectal Cancer

Whilst a detailed discussion of colorectal cancer management is outside the remit of this chapter, it is important to note that bowel resection and pelvic radiotherapy are likely to also have a significant impact on subsequent pelvic floor function including urinary function, defecatory disorders, sexual function and possibly pelvic organ prolapse. Again, the development of newer surgical and radiation techniques may limit the impact (55).

Management of Pelvic Floor Problems after Cancer

Life after cancer of any type, often signified by "ringing the bell", brings a mixture of emotions and challenges (56). Whilst the cancer treatment itself may be over, the physical and psychological impact of the cancer can remain with the patient for the rest of their life. Any factors that impact their self-confidence or quality of life, such as urinary incontinence or pelvic organ prolapse, can not only add to their anxiety but also add to this burden and potentially have a disproportionate impact. In reality the problems that present are either 1) those that have arisen as a direct result of the treatment, e.g., radiation cystitis or fistula formation, or 2) those more typical pelvic floor problems such as urinary incontinence or pelvic organ prolapse that may have been pre-existing or have developed since the cancer treatment or have been precipitated or exacerbated by the cancer treatment.

Regardless of the underlying precipitating factors, these women deserve the same attention as anyone else to their problem, with a holistic approach to their general well-being, appropriate investigations and multi-disciplinary input as appropriate. Having urinary incontinence after gynaecological cancer has a negative impact on quality of life, social interaction and sexual activity. Clinicians should also be mindful of the additional level of anxiety and loss of self-confidence that may exist in these patients.

General Principles

Positive lifestyle interventions that may help pelvic floor symptoms should be encouraged, including weight loss where appropriate, maintenance of an optimal fluid intake, avoidance of constipation, being careful with lifting techniques and minimising exposure to potential bladder irritants such as caffeine and alcohol. Pelvic floor therapies are an integral part of the management pathway and are risk-free. However, many women are unaware that pelvic floor therapy might be beneficial (57).

Dealing with Treatment Side Effects

Acute side effects of cancer treatment, by their very nature, tend to be short lived. To some extent they are predictable, and it is likely these will be largely managed by the oncology team, although specialist urology or urogynaecological help may be required if they are particularly debilitating. In some cases, it may be necessary to interrupt the radiation treatment schedule to allow the symptoms to settle down before continuing. Chronic side effects often present many years later. These can present more of a diagnostic challenge because the underlying cause may not be immediately apparent. An appropriate history should raise the index of suspicion and precipitate the relevant investigations and onward referral if necessary.

Radiation Cystitis

It should be clear from the foregoing sections that radiation cystitis is probably the most common treatment-related side effect and can be very debilitating and even life-threatening. A detailed description of its management is beyond the scope of this chapter, but a comprehensive review can be found elsewhere (24, 25, 58). In summary, whilst agents like anticholinergics and anti-inflammatory medications may help with some of the milder symptoms, the underlying problem that needs to be addressed is haematuria. This may require catheterisation, cystoscopy and clot removal, and/or bladder instillations with a variety of vasoconstricting agents such as alum, formalin, hyaluronic acid or tacrolimus. Persistent problems may require systemic therapies such as hyperbaric oxygen or ablative therapies such as fulguration or laser treatment of the bleeding points. In particularly severe cases, major intervention such as ligation of the internal iliac arteries or cystectomy and urinary diversion may have to be considered.

Fistula

Although uncommon, this severe complication may present soon after surgery or many years after the original treatment. There should be a high index of suspicion particularly for someone presenting with atypical symptoms and a past history of pelvic irradiation. A detailed description of the investigations and surgical management is beyond the scope of this chapter, but it should be obvious that with potentially fibrotic and poorly healing tissues any surgery is likely to be complex. The best results are achieved when these cases are managed within a multi-disciplinary team in specialist centres that do this type of surgery regularly.

Ureteral Strictures

Whilst these are relatively rare, they can lead to progressive obstruction of the ureter with subsequent deterioration of renal function so they need to be addressed. Initially this can be done with ureteral stents or a percutaneous nephrostomy, but if feasible, surgical correction should be performed. The nature and extent of the correction will depend on the length and position of the stricture and the overall fitness of the patient. Balloon dilatation, laser endo-uretertomy, urinary diversion or ureteral reconstruction are all possibilities (24).

Urethral Stricture

This can be a very difficult problem to manage. Urethral dilatation or urethrotomy may give temporary relief. However, because the tissues are already fibrotic, it's likely they will need to be repeated frequently which will only exacerbate the fibrosis, may cause sphincter damage and ultimately may compromise the ability to do a more definitive procedure such as a urethroplasty.

Standard Pelvic Floor Interventions

The majority of women who present with pelvic floor problems after treatment for pelvic cancer will present with the more typical symptoms (Table 5.1). Whether these symptoms have developed de novo or have been exacerbated by their cancer treatment, the approach should be the same.

Initial Assessment and Management

The initial diagnostic approach with history, examination, imaging and urodynamics should proceed as for any other woman with pelvic floor problems. If there is a significant history of radical surgery and/or radiotherapy, then particular attention should be paid to rule out the late development of the serious complications discussed earlier. Early recourse to cystoscopy and renal tract imaging may be necessary.

Basic management includes appropriate lifestyle advice regarding weight management, fluid balance, avoiding bladder stimulants (e.g. caffeine and alcohol), avoiding constipation and the use of vaginal estrogens (Chapter 4) and vaginal moisturisers. For women with intractable urinary urgency and incontinence and for those who may have radiation cystitis as well, then unfortunately standard treatments may not be appropriate or effective. Additional support may be needed such as advice regarding appropriate protection products and a "just can't wait card" (59). This is issued by the Bladder and Bowel Community and is available as a card or a phone app and is designed to show the holder has a medical condition and needs access to the toilet quickly.

Pelvic floor muscle training (PFMT) should be a standard part of any management pathway. The benefits of PFMT and other modalities such as biofeedback and electrical stimulation are well established, and they are an integral part of the management of pelvic floor problems (60, 61). The principle aims are to strengthen the pelvic floor muscles and where possible restore normal pelvic floor function. In women who have had significant pelvic surgery and or radiotherapy there may be significant underlying anatomical or fibrotic changes in the pelvic floor muscles and ligaments that may mean they are less responsive to traditional methods. However, several studies in women who have had gynaecological cancer have reported between 80% improvement in urinary incontinence symptoms with PFMT (6) and up to 90% of improvement in quality of life with multimodal PFMT treatment (62). Another study in women who had endometrial cancer found that PFMT improved pelvic floor muscle contractions and endurance in most women, and nearly 90% reported improvement in their urinary incontinence (63). Pelvic floor muscle exercises were also reported to reduce the incidence of urinary tract infection, urinary retention and pelvic discomfort after radical hysterectomy for cervical cancer (64). Ideally, PFMT could be taught before any cancer treatment, but the relatively short time scale before treatment may make this impractical. In one study pre-rehabilitation teaching had a protective effect on maintaining the intensity of the pelvic floor muscles up to one month after radiotherapy and appeared to be effective in preventing urinary incontinence (65).

Pharmacological Options

There is no reason why the normal repertoire of treatment options should not be used when indicated, such as the antimuscarinics, the β3-adrenoreceptor agonists and botulinum toxin injections. The main issue in GCS is how much radiation damage there is within the bladder and detrusor muscle. If the cause of the urgency is true overactive bladder (OAB) then it should respond normally, but if there is underlying radiation cystitis or fibrosis, then the pharmacologics mentioned may be less effective. Most of the literature relates to men after prostate cancer treatment. Given the different radiation exposure that may be employed, it's difficult to extrapolate too much; but suffice to say that after radiotherapy the bladder may not respond as well to standard treatments as one might expect in otherwise healthy cohorts. Data are relatively sparse in women, but in one observational study of 300 patients with OAB symptoms after pelvic radiotherapy, solifenacin reduced urgency, urge incontinence and nocturia over six months (66). Persistent symptoms may be very difficult to treat. Poor bladder compliance, as determined by urodynamics, appears to be associated with a lower response rate to traditional treatments for OAB such as botulinum toxin injections (58).

Surgical Interventions

Women who have had gynaecological cancer and who also present with significant stress urinary incontinence should undergo the same rigorous approach to intervention for SUI as any other urogynaecological patient with appropriate MDT discussion, the provision of appropriate patient information (67) and patient decision aids (68). The principal additional risks relate to the condition of the tissues in the retropubic space. Whatever procedure is planned, there is a risk of encountering scar tissue and fibrosis from previous radical surgery and/or radiotherapy and the additional risk of operating with sub-optimal or damaged tissues.

Again, outcome data in this cohort are limited because most studies on the management of SUI specifically exclude those who have had previous radiotherapy. There is also a persistent gender bias with most studies relating to men with urinary incontinence following prostate cancer treatment. Artificial urinary sphincter (AUS) implantation remains the "gold standard" for management of moderate to severe stress urinary incontinence in both irradiated and non-irradiated patients after prostate cancer treatment (69). Previous irradiation potentially increases the complexity of treatment because of a greater incidence of co-existing urethral stricture disease. Whilst previous pelvic irradiation seems to severely compromise the effectiveness of procedures like the AUS (70), a level of social continence similar to that of non-irradiated patients can be achieved. A number of small studies have specifically looked at SUI surgery outcomes in women who have had previous pelvic radiotherapy (71). In women, AUS after radiotherapy has a high level of erosion and failure and is not usually recommended.

Mid-urethral slings, whether with mesh or autologous tissue, remain one of the most popular surgical interventions for women with SUI worldwide. Following pelvic radiotherapy there is a risk of retropubic fibrosis and/or urethral sphincter incompetence and stricture; thus, any retropubic intervention needs to take this into account carefully in the initial decision process. Urethral pressure profilometry may help determine if there is evidence of urethral sphincter incompetence, and if so, the normal obstructive mechanism of standard mid-urethral slings may not be as effective (72). In addition, there may be a greater risk of bladder perforation with the needle placement. These concerns would seem to be borne out by the limited available data with a higher failure rate and risk of erosion (71).

Urethral bulking with its reasonable success rate, relatively minimalist intervention and low risk of serious complications (73) is potentially a more attractive option in these circumstances, but again, the data exclude women with previous radiotherapy (71). Some women may have urethral sphincter fibrosis, sometimes referred to as the drain pipe or pipe stem urethra, and in these situations the results may be less successful. In a small prospective study specifically looking at women with severe SUI and previous radiotherapy, the continence rate was 25% in women with previous radiotherapy compared to 36% in those without (74).

Similar concerns about postoperative or post-radiotherapy scarring may influence the management of women with POP. Whilst most standard procedures should be possible there may be a greater risk of visceral damage if there is significant fibrosis. Vaginal length may also have been compromised, which may increase the possibility of post-operative sexual dysfunction and pain.

As with all postmenopausal women undergoing pelvic floor surgery, vaginal estrogens can be helpful in optimising the quality of tissues prior to surgery and promoting good healing. They are rarely completely contraindicated by the previous cancer diagnosis, but their effectiveness following pelvic radiotherapy may be compromised.

Finally, it is worth considering that if a woman who presents with a pelvic cancer has pre-existing urinary incontinence or pelvic organ prolapse, is there any advantage in concurrent surgery?

Coordinated surgical intervention to address both the malignancy and pelvic floor dysfunction may enhance her postoperative quality of life and reduce the economic and quality-of-life costs of multiple surgeries (5). Concurrent surgeries have an increased incidence of minor but not serious perioperative adverse events, and one in ten planned urogynaecological procedures is either modified or abandoned during combined surgeries (75). However, the greatest challenge is probably logistical in making sure the patient has the appropriate work up for both surgeries in what will inevitably be a short time frame. Maybe this should be reserved for those who have already waited for surgical intervention and who are then diagnosed with cancer. However, even then, the prospect of postoperative radiotherapy may impact the healing process. Ultimately it would need to be assessed on a case-by-case basis.

Conclusion

Pelvic floor symptoms can be very debilitating and may well be exacerbated by the preceding cancer treatment, but with all potential interventions, the limitations of what can be achieved need to be recognised, particularly if there is significant radiation damage. Ultimately any decision on intervention should be a joint one with the relevant specialists and based on what the patient really wants to achieve in the context of their overall health (76).

Abbreviations

BMI	body mass index
CRT	conformal radiotherapy
ERBT	external beam radiotherapy
FI	faecal incontinence
GCS	gynaecological cancer survivors
IMRT	intensity-modulated radiotherapy
MR	magnetic resonance
NSRH	nerve-sparing radical hysterectomy
PFD	pelvic floor disorders
PFMT	pelvic floor muscle training
POP	pelvic organ prolapse
RH	radical hysterectomy
RT	radiotherapy
SUI	stress urinary incontinence
UUI	urinary urge incontinence
VS	vaginal stenosis

References

1. WCRF. Worldwide Cancer Data [internet]. Available from: https://www.wcrf.org/cancer-trends/worldwide-cancer-data/.
2. Rowland JH, Bellizzi KM. Cancer survivorship issues: Life after treatment and implications for an aging population. J Clin Oncol. 2014;32(24):2662–8.

3. Wu JM et al. Prevalence and trends of symptomatic pelvic floor disorders in U.S. women. Obstet Gynecol. 2014;123(1):141–8.

4. Oplawski M et al. Functional changes of the genitourinary and gastrointestinal systems before and after the treatment of endometrial cancer-a systematic review. J Clin Med. 2021;10(23):5579.

5. Thomas SG et al. Prevalence of symptomatic pelvic floor disorders among gynecologic oncology patients. Obstet Gynecol. 2013;122(5):976–80.

6. Bretschneider CE et al. Prevalence of pelvic floor disorders in women with suspected gynecological malignancy: A survey-based study. Int Urogynecol J. 2016;27:1409–14.

7. Ramaseshan AS et al. Pelvic floor disorders in women with gynecologic malignancies: A systematic review. Int Urogynecol J. 2018;29(4):459–76.

8. Chase DM et al. Assessment and significance of quality of life in women with gynecologic cancer. Future Oncol. 2010;6:1279–87.

9. Neron M et al. Impact of gynecologic cancer on pelvic floor disorder symptoms and quality of life: An observational study. Sci Rep. 2019;9:2250.

10. Donovan KA et al. Bladder and bowel symptoms in cervical and endometrial cancer survivors. Psychooncology. 2014;23:672–8.

11. Rutledge TL et al. Pelvic floor disorders and sexual function in gynecologic cancer survivors: A cohort study. Am J Obstet Gynecol. 2010;203(5):514.e1–7.

12. Manchana T et al. Long-term lower urinary tract dysfunction after radical hysterectomy in patients with early postoperative voiding dysfunction. Int Urogynecol J. 2010;21:95–101.

13. Ceccaroni M et al. Pelvic dysfunctions and quality of life after nerve-sparing radical hysterectomy: A multicenter comparative study. Anticancer Res. 2012;32(2):581–8.

14. Naik R et al. Prevalence and management of (non-fistulous) urinary incontinence in women following radical hysterectomy for early stage cervical cancer. Eur J Gynaecol Oncol. 2001;22(1):26–30.

15. Ziętek-Strobl A et al. Urogynaecological symptoms among oncological survivors and impact of oncological treatment on pelvic floor disorders and lower urinary tract symptoms: A six-month follow-up study. J Clin Med. 2020;9(9):2804.

16. Carlin GL et al. The effectiveness of surgical procedures to prevent post-hysterectomy pelvic organ prolapse: A systematic review of the literature. Int Urogynecol J. 2021;32(4):775–83.

17. Cai L et al. Pelvic floor dysfunction in gynecological cancer survivors. Eur J Obstet Gynecol Reprod Biol. 2023;288:108–13.

18. Rowland JH et al. Cancer survivorship: A new challenge in delivering quality cancer care. J Clin Oncol Off J Am Soc Clin Oncol. 2006;24:5101–4.

19. Pennycuff JF et al. Prevalence of pelvic floor disorders, associations of endocrine therapy, and surgical intervention among breast cancer survivors. Int Urogynecol J. 2022;33(9):2421–6.

20. Colombage UN et al. Experiences of pelvic floor dysfunction and treatment in women with breast cancer: A qualitative study. Support Care Cancer. 2022;30(10):8139–49.

21. Zhu L et al. Pelvic floor dysfunction after colorectal cancer treatment is related to physical and psychological health and body image: A cross-sectional study. Eur J Oncol Nurs. 2023 Dec;67:102425. doi:10.1016/j.ejon.2023.102425. Epub:2023 Oct 7. PMID:37871415.

22. Jelovsek JE et al. Pelvic organ prolapse. Lancet. 2007;369(9566):1027–38.

23. Forsgren C et al. Effects of hysterectomy on bowel function: A three-year, prospective cohort study. Dis Colon Rectum. 2007;50(8):1139–45.

24. Chorbinska J et al. Urological complications after radiotherapy-nothing ventured, nothing gained: A narrative review. Transl Cancer Res. 2021;10(2):1096–118.

25. D'Ancona CAL et al. Radiation cystitis [internet]. In: Cystitis—Updates and Challenges. IntechOpen; 2023. doi:10.5772/intechopen.111698.

26. Majeed H, Gupta V. Adverse effects of radiation therapy. In: StatPearls [internet]. Treasure Island, FL: StatPearls Publishing; 2023. Available from: https://www.ncbi.nlm.nih.gov/books/NBK563259/.

27. Dean AL. Ulceration of the urinary bladder as a late effect of radium applications to uterus. JAMA. 1927;89:1121–4.

28. Cox JD et al. Toxicity criteria of the Radiation Therapy Oncology Group (RTOG) and the European Organization for Research and Treatment of Cancer (EORTC). Int J Radiat Oncol Biol Phys. 1995;31:1341–6.

29. Common Terminology Criteria for Adverse Events (CTCAE) [internet]. National Cancer Institute, Cancer Therapy Evaluation Program. Available from: https://ctep.cancer.gov/protocolDevelopment/electronic_applications/ctc.htm#ctc_500.

30. Viswanathan AN et al. Complications of pelvic radiation in patients treated for gynecologic malignancies. Cancer. 2014;120:3870–83.

31. Parkin DE et al. Urodynamic findings following radiotherapy for cervical carcinoma. Br J Urol. 1988;61(3):213–17.

32. Georg P et al. Dose effect relationship for late side effects of the rectum and urinary bladder in magnetic resonance image-guided adaptive cervix cancer brachytherapy. Int J Radiat Oncol Biol Phys. 2012;82:653–7.

33. Roszak A et al. Incidence of radiation toxicity in cervical cancer and endometrial cancer patients treated with radiotherapy alone versus adjuvant radiotherapy. Rep Pract Oncol Radiother. 2012;17:332–8.

34. Lobo N et al. Urologic complications following pelvic radiotherapy. Urology. 2018;122:1–9.

35. Dautruche A, Delouya G. A contemporary review about the management of radiation-induced hemorrhagic cystitis. Curr Opin Support Palliat Care. 2018;12:344–50.

36. Pascoe C et al. Current management of radiation cystitis: A review and practical guide to clinical management. BJU Int. 2019;123:585–94.

37. Ma JL et al. Radiotherapy-related complications presenting to a urology department: A more common problem than previously thought? BJU Int. 2018;121(3_suppl):28–32.

38. Mendenhall WM et al. Hemorrhagic radiation cystitis. Am J Clin Oncol. 2015;38:331–6.

39. Alesawi AM et al. Radiation-induced hemorrhagic cystitis. Curr Opin Support Palliat Care. 2014;8:235–40.

40. Stamatokos M et al. Vesicovaginal fistula: Diagnosis and management. Indian J Surgery. 2014; 76(2):131–6.

41. Elliott SP, Malaeb BS. Long-term urinary adverse effects of pelvic radiotherapy. World J Urol. 2011; 29:35–41.

42. Varytė G, Bartkevičienė D. Pelvic radiation therapy induced vaginal stenosis: A review of current modalities and recent treatment advances. Medicina (Kaunas). 2021;57(4):336.

43. Ritchey M et al. Late effects on the urinary bladder in patients treated for cancer in childhood: A report from the Children's Oncology Group. Pediatr Blood Cancer. 2009;52(4):439–46.

44. Cho OH et al. Factors influencing lower urinary tract symptoms in advanced cancer patients with chemotherapy-induced peripheral neuropathy. Int Neurourol J. 2018;22(3):192–9.

45. Hazewinkel MH et al. Long-term cervical cancer survivors suffer from pelvic floor symptoms: A cross-sectional matched cohort study. Gynecol Oncol. 2010;117(2):281–6.

46. Ceccaroni M et al. Pelvic dysfunctions and quality of life after nerve-sparing radical hysterectomy: A multicenter comparative study. Anticancer Res. 2012;32(2):581–8.

47. Petersen SS et al. Rate of urologic injury with robotic hysterectomy. J Minim Invasive Gynecol. 2018;25(5):867–71.

48. Kirchheiner K et al. EMBRACE Collaborative Group. Dose-effect relationship and risk factors for vaginal stenosis after definitive radio(chemo)therapy with image-guided brachytherapy for locally advanced cervical cancer in the EMBRACE study. Radiother Oncol. 2016;118(1):160–6.

49. Nout RA et al. Long-term outcome and quality of life of patients with endometrial carcinoma treated with or without pelvic radiotherapy in the Postoperative Radiation Therapy in Endometrial Carcinoma 1 (PORTEC-1) trial. J Clin Oncol. 2011;29:1692–700.

50. De Boer SM et al. Long-term impact of endometrial cancer diagnosis and treatment on health-related quality of life and cancer survivorship: Results from the randomized PORTEC-2 trial. Int J Radiat Oncol Biol Phys. 2015;93:797–809.

51. Nosti PA et al. Symptoms of pelvic floor disorders and quality of life measures in postoperative patients with endometrial cancer. Clin Ovarian Gynecol Cancer. 2012;5(1):27–30.

52. Hopkins MP et al. Radical vulvectomy: The decision for the incision. Cancer. 1993;72(3):799–803.

53. Hampl M et al. The risk of urinary incontinence after partial urethral resection in patients with anterior vulvar cancer. Eur J Obstet Gynecol Reprod Biol. 2011;154(1):108–12.

54. Hoffman MS et al. A comparative study of radical vulvectomy and modified radical vulvectomy for the treatment of invasive squamous cell carcinoma of the vulva. Gynecol Oncol. 1992;45(2):192–7.

55. Giglia MD, Stein SL. Overlooked long-term complications of colorectal surgery. Clin Colon Rectal Surg. 2019 May;32(3):204–11.

56. Bell RJ. Ringing the bell and then falling off a cliff . . . life after cancer. Climacteric. 2019;22(6):533–4.

57. Lindgren A et al. Experiences of incontinence and pelvic floor muscle training after gynecologic cancer treatment. Support Care Cancer. 2017;25(1):157–66.

58. Bosch R et al. Can radiation-induced lower urinary tract disease be ameliorated in patients treated for pelvic organ cancer: ICI-RS 2019. Neurourol Urodyn. 2020;39:S148–55.

59. Bladder and Bowel UK. Just Can't Wait Card. Available from: https://www.bbuk.org.uk/just-cant-wait-cards/.

60. Dumoulin C et al. Keeping the pelvic floor healthy. Climacteric. 2019;22(3):257–62.

61. Rutledge TL et al. A pilot randomized control trial to evaluate pelvic floor muscle training for urinary incontinence among gynecologic cancer survivors. Gynecol Oncol. 2014;132(1):154–8.

62. Cyr MP et al. Feasibility, acceptability and effects of multimodal pelvic floor physical therapy for gynecological cancer survivors suffering from painful sexual intercourse: A multicenter prospective interventional study. Gynecol Oncol. 2020;159(3):778–84.

63. Bernard S et al. An in-home rehabilitation program for the treatment of urinary incontinence symptoms in endometrial cancer survivors: A single-case experimental design study. Int Urogynecol J. 2021;32:2947–57.

64. Zong S et al. Effect of Kegel pelvic floor muscle exercise combined with clean intermittent self-catheterization on urinary retention after radical hysterectomy for cervical cancer. Pak J Med Sci. 2022;38(3 Part-I):462–8.

65. Sacomori C et al. Pre-rehabilitation of the pelvic floor before radiation therapy for cervical cancer: A pilot study. Int Urogynecol J. 2020;31(11):2411–18.

66. Jaszczyński J et al. Post-irradiation bladder syndrome after radiotherapy of malignant neoplasm of small pelvis organs: An observational, non-interventional clinical study assessing VESIcare®/Solifenacin treatment results. Med Sci Monit. 2016;22:2691–8.

67. British Society of Urogynecology. Patient Information Leaflets [internet]. Available from: https://bsug.org.uk/pages/for-patients/bsug-patient-information-leaflets/154.

68. NICE. Surgery for Stress Urinary Incontinence [internet]. Available from: https://www.nice.org.uk/guidance/ng123/resources/surgery-for stress-urinary-incontinence-patient-decision-aid-pdf-6725286110.

69. Sathianathen NJ et al. Outcomes of artificial urinary sphincter implantation in the irradiated patient. BJU Int. 2014;113(4):636–41.

70. Torrey R et al. Radiation history affects continence outcomes after advance transobturator sling placement in patients with post-prostatectomy incontinence. Urology. 2013;82(3):713–17.

71. Dobberfuhl AD. Evaluation and treatment of female stress urinary incontinence after pelvic radiotherapy. Neurourol Urodyn. 2018;1–11.

72. Carlson K et al. 2024 Canadian urological association guideline: Female stress urinary incontinence. Can Urol Assoc J. 2024 Apr;18(4):83–102.

73. Kirchin V et al. Urethral injection therapy for urinary incontinence in women. Cochrane Database Syst Rev. 2017;7:CD003881.

74. Krhut J et al. Treatment of stress urinary incontinence using polyacrylamide hydrogel in women after radiotherapy: 1-year follow-up. Int Urogynecol J. 2016;27:301–5.

75. Davidson ERW et al. Perioperative adverse events in women undergoing concurrent urogynecologic and gynecologic oncology surgeries for suspected malignancy. Int Urogynecol J. 2019;30(7):1195–201.

76. Robinson D et al. What do women want? Interpretation of the concept of cure. J Pelvic Med Surg. 2003;9:273–7.

Chapter 6

Sexual Health and Intimacy

Claudine Domoney and Elle Sein

Introduction

The diagnosis of malignancy challenges many aspects of an individual's perception of existence. The journey of diagnosis, treatment and survivorship is individual and dependent on ongoing support, both personal and professional. The impact of this journey can be mitigated by an understanding of the varied and sometimes unpredictable consequences of treatment by healthcare professionals, the patient and their partners, family and friends. The influence of various treatments for cancers on body image, sexual health and fertility needs careful discussion.

As the incidence of cancer increases worldwide—approximately 40.5% of men and women will be diagnosed with cancer in their lifetime (1), high numbers of cancer survivors need ongoing specialist care. In 2022, there were 20 million new cases of cancer and more than 385,000 new cases in the UK (2). In women, breast cancer is the leading cause of cancer death (3). Although the majority of cancers in women occur during the postmenopausal phase, a significant minority are diagnosed in childhood or during their reproductive lifetime. The proportion of cancers directly affecting sexual organs is much higher in women than men. Yet the focus of sexual health care for female survivors is demonstrably less. Body image and fertility potential are closely linked to sexual functioning, particularly in younger age groups, but under researched.

Sexual health as determined by the WHO refers to physical, emotional, mental and social wellbeing related to sexuality and is fundamental to overall health and well-being, quality of life and social status, not the absence of disease, dysfunction or infirmity (4). A cancer diagnosis will impact physical, emotional, mental and social wellbeing, with effects on sexuality, sexual functioning, body image and the potential impact on fertility being components of the complexity of these interactions. For some women, a cancer diagnosis may also mean a diagnosis of infertility. The subsequent treatment plan will be dependent on a negotiation of these factors by the individual with their healthcare professionals and needs to be individualised. It is therefore incumbent on those involved in caring for these people to facilitate an understanding of the interactions on an individual basis.

Prevalence of Sexual Problems

Sexual problems are highly prevalent in women (approximately 41%) from a meta-analysis of premenopausal women (5), but estimates vary depending on the population, the questionnaires used

DOI: 10.1201/9781032631028-6

and assessment of distress associated with sexual issues, which includes lack of arousal and desire, orgasmic difficulty and pain (for further classification details see the International Classification of Diseases-10 and/or the Diagnostic and Statistical Manual of Mental Disorders [DSM-V] of the American Psychiatric Association). Cancer treatments which affect gynaecological function, including hormonal disruption, fertility potential, the ability to carry a pregnancy and bladder and bowel function, will likely have long-term consequences on sexual functioning. The overall psychological effect of a cancer diagnosis and the subsequent treatment and recovery will depend on baseline and historical experiences. Menopausal transition, induced surgically or medically, superimposed on poor physical, mental and sexual health often causes significant negative symptoms with detrimental effects on function and quality of life. These multifactorial and interacting complexities can be difficult to ascertain quantitatively and qualitatively in different patient groups with varied assessment instruments. However, it is clear that women have significant ongoing sexual health concerns that persist from diagnosis to long-term follow-up. Patient education and information are imperative to allow patients to consider options for treatment of these distressing symptoms.

Screening and Monitoring Change in Sexual Function/Dysfunction

Simple screening questions by healthcare professionals in a general population have been shown to be as effective as a long interview with a sexual therapist (6) and could be adapted to consultations at different stages of diagnosis and treatment of cancer. Baseline sexual functioning may be compromised prior to diagnosis due to anxiety caused by presenting symptoms such as irregular or postcoital bleeding. This has been documented amongst those having positive HPV screening and cervical treatment (7).

Questions used to screen for sexual problems (see the following) may be adapted for subsequent consultations (6):

1. Are you sexually active? (Or are you in a sexual relationship?)
2. Are there any problems?
3. Do you have any pain (or bleeding) with intercourse?

Patient-reported outcome measures that aim to assess meaningful or clinically relevant change may be particularly helpful in sensitive areas including sexual function. However there are many provisos when choosing the appropriate questionnaire: the length of recall, number of items/questions, and sensitivity for measuring a relevant outcome in a specific patient group. Generic questionnaires such as the Changes in Sexual Functioning Questionnaire (CSFQ) (8) were designed to measure illness and medication effects on sexual functioning whereas the freely available condition-specific instrument Female Sexual Function Index (FSFI) (9) was validated initially to detect arousal disorder, then orgasmic and desire disorders. The FSFI is often used to determine those with and without sexual dysfunction. Disease-specific questionnaires will be validated in persons with a particular condition and are designed to detect change within that population, so may limit comparison to other groups. The Female Sexual Distress Scale (FSDS) may elucidate the clinical relevance of sexual dysfunction. The European Organisation for Research and Treatment of Cancer (EORTC) (10) has created questionnaires (some, but not all, validated) pertaining to people with specific cancers. Questionnaires may also be heteronormative in their design and validation, which should also be acknowledged. The questionnaires widely used are reviewed by

Jeffrey et al. 2016 (11). General health and medication use may also impact sexual functioning independently. Other scales can measure body image (see later) and overall mental health (e.g., Hospital Anxiety and Depression scale, HADS).

Consultation Differences between Men and Women with Cancer Having Sexual Concerns

There are many studies of the difference between men and women undergoing cancer treatment being asked about sexual concerns. Up to 80% of men having prostate cancer treatment were asked about sex compared with 33% of women with breast cancer (12). Taylor et al. 2020 (13) suggested 87% of patients in a radiotherapy clinic felt their treatment impacted sexual function but only 28% reported being asked. Men were significantly more likely to be asked about sexual health by their healthcare professionals compared with women (53% versus 22%). The gender identity and sexual orientation of cancer survivors will also hugely impact the delivery and reception of care, but is variably recorded. It has more recently become an expanding field of research (see later).

Sexual Function According to Hormonal Status

Studies of sexual function and body image in naturally menopausal women can be contradictory and vary according to stage of menopause. The impact of menopausal symptoms on general health including sleep, wellbeing and libido in addition to the dyspareunia of genitourinary syndrome of menopause, caused by oestrogen deficiency, is well recognised amongst physiologically menopausal women. Studies in cancer survivorship quality of life, body image and sexual problems are also variable but generally associated with deterioration. The degree of distress caused by induced menopause may be more significant in premenopausal women. As discussed, the availability of disease-specific sexual function questionnaires may be limited and also not comparable to the general population, so of variable value. Comparison of studies for treatment interventions during the timeline of cancer diagnosis and treatment is therefore challenging. Prior menopausal and fertility status contributes to intimacy and childbearing concerns, but the feeling of loss is individual. Tackling the potential future consequences for a child treated for cancer with chemotherapy, radiotherapy and/or surgery, causing fertility compromise, perceived mutilation and potential self-esteem and body image problems, poses additional ethical complications.

Impact of Cancer on Sexual Health

Pelvic cancers including vulval, cervical, endometrial and ovarian in addition to colorectal cancers will have a direct impact on the physical and therefore psychological context of sexual activity. However, management of other non-pelvic cancers, particularly breast, but commonly haematological malignancies and others which, by nature of chemotherapeutic or radiotherapy interventions, will compromise the hypothalamic-pituitary-ovarian (HPO) axis, directly affects sexual functioning and fertility potential. The physical effects of surgery, radiotherapy, chemotherapy and subsequent menopausal/temporary oestrogen deficiency symptoms alter the psychosomatic functioning of an individual. Sexual activity is the ultimate psychosomatic activity, involving both mind and body. The presentation of sexual difficulties can be unpredictable and individual-specific, dependent on their background and baseline functioning. Because sexual difficulties may manifest acutely, at intermediate follow-up and/or long-term follow-up, it is imperative that sexual health is a routine part of consultation questioning. Symptoms may present overtly or covertly. Physical examination may also be 'a moment of truth' when the subconscious can present the conflict in returning to 'normal' during the survivorship journey. Clinicians looking after cancer survivors should have training in recognising which women need referral for psychosexual problems and, where feasible, brief training in this area (14). It is common to recognise the breast, vagina and body that is no longer a place of pleasure but of medical examination.

A return to sexual health is an important sign of recovery in those partnered and not partnered. Currently, low- and middle-income countries are less likely to consider sexual outcomes of importance and may be considered only in the context of family relationships (15). The range of treatment options can be more limited and less individually personalised. There may be cultural taboos rgarding diagnosis and interventions in addition to affordable access to multiprofessional care. However, the demand for information is still present and necessary in all populations, so should be contextually tailored. Since women suffer more cancers directly affecting their sexual organs, a manifesto for preservation of sexual function is paramount for maintenance of wellbeing and relationships (16). This manifesto highlights the importance of establishing evidence-based approaches for addressing sexual health in cancer survivors.

Ascertaining whether the cancer treatments and their consequences have caused sexual dysfunction rather than the common sexual problems of the general population is challenging when the training of healthcare professionals in this area is limited. Seeing these problems through the 'medical gaze' of a cancer survivor may normalise the complexities but also may shield the patient from receiving routine care that persons without a cancer diagnosis may receive. Conversations about sexual health, intimacy and fertility at all stages of cancer diagnosis and treatment should be available for the vast majority of those undergoing it. Given its multifaceted dimensions, a multidisciplinary team is required to provide appropriate services. Detecting difficulties in clinical practice with simple screening questions can be tailored to the specific stage of diagnosis and treatment. Subsequently appropriate supportive or specialist care can then be offered. Acknowledging its importance even if help is declined is important. This 'permission giving' encourages the patient to raise these issues again in the future when they wish. It also recognises sexual functioning as a valued feature of recovery. There are also multiple support groups that patients can access once they have been discharged back to their primary care providers if they have ongoing issues with sexual health and intimacy. These can be accessed through Cancer Research UK and patients can be signposted to these resources by GPs.

Impact of Treatment Interventions

On General Health

The diagnosis and treatment of cancers are widely recognised to cause fatigue, depression and anxiety in addition to many other multisystem complaints that impact quality of life. Although many survivors of cancer treatments over five years report good general health, they demonstrate ongoing physical and psychological effects. Age and income in addition to being female may contribute to this (17). However, the reframing of life goals and sense of purpose that may enhance existence is little studied. Predicting those at risk of long-term sequelae and supportive care from healthcare professionals may improve quality of life during survivorship.

On the Hypothalamic-Pituitary-Ovarian (HPO) Axis

Surgical menopause with removal of the ovaries is a common procedure for pelvic tumours. Adjacent surgical procedures may induce ovarian insufficiency through vascular compromise. Chemotherapy and radiotherapy for pelvic and nonpelvic tumours can accelerate ovarian failure. Diagnosis of menopausal status or primary ovarian insufficiency (POI) in the under-40 age group is however not straightforward. For some treatments, there is a possibility of recovery of function, although this is currently unpredictable. The ESHRE definition of POI includes four consecutive cycles with menstrual irregularity and a raised FSH of 40 iU/L on two occasions with more than a month interval (18). This will identify those women who require hormone therapy discussions but is not helpful for indicating possible recovery.

Anti-Mullerian hormone (AMH) may be used as a surrogate marker for ovarian reserve but reference ranges are wide and of limited clinical specificity. AMH is a glycoprotein produced in the granulosa cells of ovarian follicles independent of the menstrual cycle. It suppresses the primordial follicle pool, so with its loss during destruction of larger follicles by chemotherapy, the primordial follicle pool is recruited, then activated; but this finite pool is then depleted and can no longer replace the active follicles (which are more easily damaged by chemotherapy). Direct damage to the primordial follicles and ovarian tissues will also contribute to ovarian functioning via vasoconstriction, inhibition of angiogenesis and follicular apoptosis and death, but may be recoverable. The primordial follicular pool is therefore more relatively protected and explains why childhood cancer survivors may have a lower but ongoing fertility potential. Measurement of FSH, LH and oestradiol may indicate recovery.

There are more significant data regarding the impact of older chemotherapy agents, but this will depend on the baseline fertility status of the individual. Some chemotherapy agents such as alkylating agents have a more toxic effect and therefore may influence treatment decision making. This will clearly vary from prepubertal girls to women of childbearing potential and those later in their reproductive years. There is no clear process for detecting ovarian reserve or aging. Measuring ovarian potential currently relies on antral follicle count (by ultrasound scan) and AMH levels, which are surrogate markers for ovarian reserve. These are better used for predicting success in oocyte retrieval, so the limitations are clear. However, it is suggested that AMH can be used for monitoring ovarian damage during chemotherapy and determining differential effects of newer therapies (19).

On Quality of Life (QoL) and Sexual Functioning

The WHO definition of quality of life is 'an individual's perception of their position in life in the context of the culture and value systems in which they live and in relation to their goals, expectations, standards and concerns' (20). Sexuality is defined as not only the ability to engage in sexual activity but also as components of femininity or masculinity, reproductive ability, appearance and sexual functional capacity (21). Sexual functioning is the ability to engage in sexual activity, intercourse or self-stimulation and includes components of desire, arousal, lubrication, orgasm and satisfaction in addition to pain. However, different researchers use different definitions within studies. Cancer treatment will affect QoL psychologically, physically and/or hormonally.

Although surgery involving removal of gynaecological organs and bowel can compromise the adjacent structures so may determine the extent of sexual impact, the role of each sexual organ in sexual pleasure is variable. This includes breast cancer surgery and reconstruction. Advances in surgical technique with laparoscopic and robotic approaches have reported improved outcomes for malignancies, but these surgical options are not universally available. The data will guide surgical oncologists' approach, but will always need individualisation. Although it appears that minimal access surgery will facilitate more rapid recovery and lower depression scores, the long-term impact may differ.

Early-stage endometrial and ovarian disease is amenable to endoscopic approaches with improved outcome for body image and quality of life, although the sexual outcomes are more varied depending on the structure of the study, questionnaires used to assess and surgical techniques. With respect to endometrial cancer, laparoscopy fared better overall than open operative management, and vaginal brachytherapy better than external beam radiotherapy (22). High body mass index was associated with poorer overall quality of life and more fatigue. Sexual function was related to age at diagnosis, time since diagnosis and consulting a physician before resuming sexual activity.

Little is known about the psychosexual impact of ovarian cancer. This may reflect poorer prognosis due to late presentation, with only 15% diagnosed at early stages and 46% five-year survival rate. Surgeries, which may be multiple, and chemotherapy (less often radiotherapy) have different mechanisms of negative effects—endocrine, direct physical and psychological. Up to 86% of patients treated for epithelial ovarian cancers report a sexual issue (23), yet these are infrequently addressed.

A retrospective cervical cancer study suggested greater dissection had increased ongoing negative sexual and quality of life effects compared with less extensive surgery and adjuvant therapies (24). Their data suggest cervical cancer survivors have the worst quality of life due to their young age and the long-term consequences of therapy. The Laparoscopic Approach to Cervical Cancer (LACC) trial determined that in cervical cancers over 2 cm in size, those having an open approach had improved survival outcomes (25) although this resulted in worse sexual functioning and quality of life (26) in addition to poorer body image (27). Another group suggested that surgical technique should not be standardised given the significant impact on predominantly young women with cervical cancer (28). Therefore, the determination of route of surgery requires consideration beyond the literature data. The aim is not a fight with pathology only but the goal of optimising quality of life, particularly given the increased survival after treatment.

On the Urogenital Tract

The urogenital tract is hormonally and physically sensitive to treatments for many cancers. Minimising the impact of surgery with assessment of newer techniques by use of patient-reported outcome measures is crucial. Oestrogen deficiency caused by ovarian disruption affects all tissue functioning in premenopausal women. This is mediated by changes in the vaginal and bladder mucosa, and pelvic floor. The bladder may develop increased overactivity, more incontinence and recurrent UTIs. If the bowel is similarly affected, this is even more impactful. Chemotherapeutic agents have differential direct toxic effects on mucosa affecting bladder and vaginal responses. The physical effects of radiotherapy will change over time and induce longer-term consequences. Chemotherapy may also result in negative consequences via ovarian damage, and therefore oestrogen deficiency. These effects may be mitigated with shielding or transposition of the ovaries from the radiation field and in younger women inducing medical menopause with GnRH agonists may partly reduce chemotherapeutic ovarian toxicity. This is discussed in detail in another chapter.

Radiotherapy (for bladder, gynaecological and lower bowel cancers) can cause inflammation, oedema, fibrosis, necrosis and similar effects on neighbouring pelvic organs, and as previously discussed, ovarian failure with its sequelae. These are acute, intermediate and long-term in nature—some reversal may be expected. With brachytherapy implants and during the acute phase, penetrative activities should be avoided. Chemotherapy has systemic effects, and includes menopausal symptoms mediated through the impact on the HPO axis (although many side effects of chemotherapy may mimic oestrogen deficiency); these may be temporary. Vaginal dryness, mucosal ulcers and suppression of the immune system may encourage other infections of the genital tract. Discharge (both vaginal and rectal) and bleeding compromises sexual function. The reduction in intercourse may perpetuate these problems, both physically and psychosexually. Maintenance of vaginal patency after radiotherapy, particularly brachytherapy, for pelvic tumours will encourage ongoing penetrative sexual activity.

The impact of all therapeutic interventions for gynaecological cancers on bladder and bowel symptoms cannot be over emphasised (29)—both direct and indirect, causing pain, bladder and bowel overactivity and incontinence, which has been noted to increase the negative impact on body image and sexual function, particularly in those of a younger age.

On Body Image

Following the diagnosis of cancer and the treatment that follows, women will experience changes to their body and often side effects from treatment. These include surgical scarring, loss of organs (breasts, uterus, cervix, ovaries) and the impact of entering menopause, urinary and bowel symptoms, vaginal dryness and chronic pain (30, 31). These physical changes can lead to the perception of a changed female body and 'body image'.

The term body image has many definitions within psychosocial oncology. It can be described as a 'multifaceted construct that involves perceptions, thoughts, feelings and behaviours related to the entire body and its functioning (30). It is the sum of several identity factors, emotions, feelings and actions (32) and can reflect the way in which one views and experiences their body subjectively (33). The National Cancer Institute defines body image as 'the way a person thinks about his or her body and how it looks to others' (34).

Cash developed a cognitive-behavioural model of body image, with an emphasis on viewing body image as a complex phenomenon with a number of interrelated variables (35). The model is based on the concepts of 'body image evaluation' and 'body image investment'. Body image evaluation relates to the degree of satisfaction with one's body image and the discrepancy between self-perceived and desired body characteristics. This relates to the role of cultural socialisation, societal views on women and the role of 'femininity'. The female organs have historically been regarded as the core of 'femininity' and may still be considered key in gender identity to society. This contributes to 'objectification theory' that states that women are sexualised by society, and the body is seen and judged in a sexual context (36). In addition, the 'event' of cancer and its treatment can be seen to activate a self-evaluation of one's physical appearance and hence their body image (35).

White, working on Cash's model, emphasises the subjective nature of body image and postulates that we must consider the woman's perspective regardless of the objective appearance of bodily changes and function to the healthcare professional (37). Somatisation can be present, referring to psychological distress in which personal distress is expressed through physical symptoms in the absence of any underlying organic cause (38). Body image concerns can be viewed on a spectrum or continuum, that small interventions or acknowledgement may reduce avoidance of intimate relationships and subsequent isolation and loneliness.

The prevalence of body image issues in cancer is hard to assess, with little evidence in the literature. Most research on body image in cancer has been conducted in breast cancer. Up to 30% women following treatment for breast cancer have concerns over their body image (39). Women who suffer with gynaecological cancers also express negative body image and sexual functioning, which can lead to distancing from intimate relationships (40). This often results from a combination of physical symptoms (urinary and faecal incontinence, menopausal symptoms including vaginal dryness and low libido), and the psychological impact of a cancer diagnosis and requirement for surgery and other therapies. The removal of the uterus can be significant in a woman's identity (41). Many cultures place huge value on women being defined by the ability to bear children. Therefore it follows that women are more likely to experience body image concerns if of reproductive age at diagnosis. Surgical complications and traumatic experiences during treatment magnify this. These factors are often unavoidable, but it is important to recognise when considering the holistic care provided by the MDT.

Responses to body image distress, which include avoidance strategies such as refraining from intimacy, sexual activity and relationships, result in lower emotional wellbeing (42), anxiety and depression. Women may benefit from talking about body image and the resulting sequelae, including the sexual dysfunction and intimacy issues that can develop post cancer. Healthcare professionals must ask about body image—being open and responsive may give them the confidence to talk about these concerns. Being realistic about bodily changes post treatment can reduce shame and disappointment. These include the bodily changes secondary to neurological damage, reconstructive flaps with consequent changes in sensation, hair loss and oestrogen deficiency. Addressing the experience of treatment may allow reframing of thoughts through CBT and behavioural/psychological interventions.

A paper reviewing 121 studies regarding body image, sexuality and sexual functioning with respect to cervical and uterine cancers (43) used both quantitative and qualitative data. The vast majority investigated sexual functioning (n = 72) with few focusing alone on sexuality (n = 8) and body image (n = 3) but 38 had more than one component and 6 all three aspects. This paper defined body image as comprising emotional and behavioural response to perceived appearance, sexuality and femininity based on self-perception rather than the perceptions of others, although this does encompass a cultural perspective. Younger age groups, those with bladder and bowel dysfunction, in addition to those with recurrence, were most affected.

Of interest in this paper were significant differences in body image and sexuality in lower- and middle-income countries in comparison to more developed countries, where the former were more focused on intimacy and gender, in comparison to the latter in whom body image and changing perception of femininity were expressed more frequently. Some of these disparities were noted between ethnic groups within the United States. It was determined there were also discrepancies in information provided with respect to these issues, although patients wanted to have these conversations. The lack of information regarding body image and sexuality, however, was correlated, and predicted sexual functioning.

Focusing on body image and sexuality may help direct care to those who are more likely to be compromised due to early expressions of negative impact, perhaps secondary to baseline functioning. Many patients expressed the desire for more information on the impact of the diagnosis and treatment, having not received it.

Stoma Formation

Temporary or permanent stoma formation impacts mental as well as sexual health. Although it has been reported that there is no difference between cancer and non-cancer groups, intimacy issues are significant (44). Up to half of patients sexually active before their stoma formation did not resume sexual activity. However for those who did, most were satisfied. Sensitively discussing resumption of physical relationships and practical issues with the patient and their intimate partners will assist with longer-term sexual health (45).

On Fertility

The impact on fertility of cancer depends on site, type, staging and treatment required, in addition to age and menopausal status. Therapeutic intervention is determined depending on fertility desires which may in turn be related to age, previous pregnancies and partner status. The age and baseline fertility status will help direct counselling, but there is evidence that external fertility counselling aside from that of the oncologist may be helpful and associated with less regret, particularly in younger patients (46). However, the perception of delay in treatment, the impact on psychological health, risk of a subsequent pregnancy, vertical transmission of cancer genes and cost or access to services may limit fertility preservation conversations and interventions. There is evidence that given a choice, many more would seek this information than receive it (47). However fertility preservation techniques currently available are limited despite ongoing improvement and for many are still experimental with low ongoing live pregnancy capability.

Cancer-related fertility concerns have been described as the double burden, involving not only fertility but changing sexual intimacy and feelings of inadequacy with forming new relationships. Considering fertility as a significant concern when compared to the 'privilege of survival', survivors may often feel they cannot raise it, although for young patients there is evidence this is one of the most difficult long-term consequences (47). Making decisions about potential childbearing may be seen as a sign of having the options of people living without a history of cancer, and couples with coping strategies that include the 'we disease' approach, i.e. a joint approach to the complexities of cancer survivorship, have increased relationship satisfaction with reduced distress (48). Overprotective behaviours and disengaged avoidance may reduce the ability of the patient to share their feelings with consequent reduced relationship satisfaction and poor mental health (49). Ussher's group therefore recommend that couples are seen together and that partners are involved in fertility discussions (50).

Radiotherapy that may preserve fertility (total body, abdominal and some low dose pelvic irradiation) still impacts pregnancy such that there is an observable increase in adverse outcomes including miscarriage, preterm labour and low birth weight for gynaecological and childhood cancers, with abdominal radiotherapy increasing the risk of gestational diabetes, anaemia and hypertension (51). Total body irradiation increases the risks for donor oocyte pregnancies which would usually be related to the donor age, implying an effect on placentation (via the endometrial receptivity) and the potential for uterine support (via vascularity and myometrium) (52). Specialist obstetric support is warranted for these cancer survivors.

Management of Fertility Preservation in Women

The current techniques for oocyte preservation, although much improved over the last decade, still depend on the quality of egg retrieved, in turn dependent on the age of the patient, and the delicate process of vitrification/freezing then successful thawing (around 85%) of the delicate oocyte, which results in a low live birth rate (although currently equivalent to fresh embryo pregnancy rates).

Egg freezing, which requires stimulation of the ovaries with sex steroid hormones over a period of a few weeks, although not dependent on time of menstrual cycle, may not be successful. There are also the risks of ovarian hyperstimulation syndrome, hormonal stimulation of an oestrogen-sensitive tumour, risks associated with the egg retrieval itself, possible seeding of malignant cells, and delay in starting primary cancer treatment.

The aromatase inhibitor letrozole reduces oestrogen levels in the body by blocking androgen conversion to oestrogen and has been used during ovarian stimulation in oestrogen receptor-positive breast cancer patients because it does not appear to affect egg yield.

Embryo freezing is more successful but requires a partner who consents to preservation and continues to consent when the opportunity for implantation arises at an appropriate time after treatment (often several years). The legal status of ownership of the embryo varies worldwide, and the religious and moral implications surrounding creation of embryos limit its use for some. It is also menstrual cycle-dependent. However currently the pregnancy rate in the UK with frozen embryos is 36% with a 30% birth rate compared with a lower rate for fresh embryos which would be more comparable after successful egg thawing with ICSI (intra-cytoplasmic sperm insemination). There are differences with age as well as ethnic variation in pregnancy rates.

Ovarian tissue cryopreservation is still in its infancy with few reports of live ongoing pregnancies. However, the option to preserve tissue removed laparoscopically can be discussed and is likely of importance to children and younger people undergoing cancer treatment, although due to the protection of the primordial follicles, they may be at lower risk of permanent fertility cessation depending on treatment.

Women requiring pelvic radiation may be offered transposition of the ovaries or oophoropexy whereby the ovaries are fixed as high as possible on the pelvic sidewall, usually by a laparoscopic approach or as part of the primary surgery (open or laparoscopic), protecting them from the radiation field. Ovarian shielding during the radiation process may be an alternative option for some.

The use of gonadotropin releasing hormone (GnRH) agonists to protect the ovaries by inducing a postmenopausal state or 'medical menopause' makes the ovaries less susceptible to the menstrual cycle changes from the hypothalamic-pituitary-ovarian (HPO) axis. This has improved the number of pregnancies and ovarian and menstrual dysfunction in some studies, although others have indicated no change in menstrual status, AMH or FSH levels.

Although there are various guidelines, the consistency of their application with respect to discussion of fertility preservation is variable. The barriers to this have been cited as time, knowledge, opinion on professional responsibility, lack of written information and variable access to fertility specialists (53). A Dutch study identified that online written information and patient decision making aids would be the most helpful for them and their populations. Although access to pre-treatment counselling and establishment of fertility potential may be limited, this may significantly impact the journey of survivorship for these patients. Consensus recommendations should be developed as a baseline for all cancer services.

Impact on Menstruation

Gonad-preserving treatments may still have an impact on menstruation, inducing disturbed cycles with heavier, lighter or more unpredictable flow, symptoms associated with low oestrogen including night sweats, hot flushes, poor sleep, low mood and cognitive decline, in addition to an impact on sexual function. The likelihood of these occurring or persisting is proportional to the ovarian age or reserve. The amount of radiation causing amenorrhoea is significantly lower for a woman over 40 than a younger woman. Although the probability of recovery from these symptoms in different age groups has been documented for many chemotherapy agents and some radiotherapy regimes, little is known about the impact of newer targeted therapies and immunotherapy. There is a need for these endpoints to be added to all clinical trials, particularly in young people.

Impact on Pregnancy

It is well documented that radiation to the uterus can cause changes in its future potential for successful pregnancy, including damage to the vascular and muscular tissues. Total body radiation increases the risk of miscarriage, preterm labour and low birth weight although lower doses locally may have less impact. Radiotherapy to the ovary will have a dose-dependent destructive impact on the primordial follicles and oocytes. The potential for gamete damage perpetuated via chromosome changes to ongoing pregnancies is less well documented but another concern for survivors. Surgery may be modified to preserve fertility potential depending on degree of risk, or a plan for completion surgery at a later date, depending on the individual characteristics. The radical trachelectomy for cervical cancer was developed to preserve the possibility of ongoing pregnancy albeit with a higher risk of pregnancy loss and pre-term labour. Early-stage endometrial cancer, borderline and stage 1 ovarian tumours may be managed with conservative surgery for individuals with particular fertility wishes after careful multidisciplinary discussion.

Impact of Cervical Cancer Screening

Information regarding HPV testing as a screening test, and HPV's link to cervical and anal cancers, may reduce the persistent psychosexual impact that has been demonstrated. A systematic review detailed the negative psychosexual impact of a diagnosis of HPV infection and colposcopic examination, even without a diagnosis of malignancy (54). Although there were some inconsistencies, most studies indicated an impact on psychosexual outcomes, with some lasting for over two years. This highlights the need for patient-centred information and psychological follow-up. The success of HPV testing and vaccination has led to a significant decline in incidence of HPV-related disease and an improvement in survival rates globally (55), but uptake and gender-neutral access still needs significant improvement to reduce future post-treatment long-term effects (56) and education to reduce the fear associated with HPV, perceived as a sexually transmitted infection progressing to cancer. For those with treated cancer and those without, unscheduled bleeding, postcoital or not, is an ominous symptom that impacts healthy sexual lives. This association with sexual activity can lead to a belief that sex may aggravate the cancer and/or treatment failure despite it being a common consequence of treatment (57).

Impact of Cancers on Sexual Health

Cervical Cancer

The surgical data has been briefly discussed in previous sections and warrants ongoing studies as new techniques are introduced. Longitudinal data observing the treatment impact of chemotherapy, radiotherapy and brachytherapy, compared with surgery, indicated an improvement over time (28) despite being worse with respect to sexual function in the short term (58), although those treated without surgery generally had more advanced disease. Sexual functioning and quality of life declined significantly after treatment for cervical cancer irrespective of stage and therapeutic intervention. Overall, there was no difference with radical trachelectomy, open radical hysterectomy or a laparoscopic approach. However, there are differences in body image and recovery. The specific components of reduced sexual function are different although the studies are heterogenous (59). This systematic review examines data from 18 studies investigating quality of life and sexual function after treatment of cervical cancer. All studies showed a decrease in sexual function in patients with cervical cancer, but the reasons for this sexual dysfunction were varied, related to physical issues, depression and body image concerns. The most important factors were stage of disease and the therapeutic intervention, with the combination of surgery and adjuvant therapy affecting depression and sexual function most, with least recovery (60). The most frequent causes of female sexual dysfunction were negative impact on quality of life, depression, loss of libido, anxiety and impact of surgery on body image. Physical issues, if addressed prior to treatment, may be more susceptible to intervention by anticipating a psychological impact. Education of patients and open discussion are likely to be useful interventions and in many studies have been noted to be lacking.

Endometrial Cancer

With respect to endometrial cancer, most studies have examined surgery alone versus surgery and radiotherapy. Surgery alone produces fewer long-lasting consequences and may be comparable to hysterectomised age-matched controls in the postmenopausal group. There may appear to be less impact of brachytherapy on overall quality of life compared with external beam radiotherapy but there are risks of vaginal stenosis and adhesions in addition to urethral and bladder scarring, which need to be proactively addressed. The impact on sexual functioning depends very much on pre-treatment activity—studies have indicated that lower levels of pre-treatment activity and raised BMI can predict poorer ongoing function (61). This population is an older group in comparison to those diagnosed with cervical cancer, so may have lower activity rates overall, but the opportunity for open discussion should be given. Modification of treatment according to tissue damage and recurrence rate can be increasingly discussed with patients when there is a dialogue about function and quality of life after treatment for cancer.

Vulval Cancer

Vulval cancer is a rare malignancy but well recognised as having a significant sexual impact and worsening quality of life (62). Surgery and radiotherapy reduce sensation and increase vaginal and urethral narrowing with additional lymphoedema. This may produce a perception of mutilation to a part that many may not name or be familiar with anatomically. There also appears to be little recovery over time and may be perceived as an 'old ladies' disease'.

Bladder Cancer

The data with respect to bladder cancer is poor for women with small numbers comparing surgery with radiotherapy, using a variety of patient-reported outcome measures (PROMs). Those sexually active prior to diagnosis and treatment had a significant reduction in desire, but it is not clear whether modifications in surgery or other adjuvant therapies will modify this (63).

Bowel Cancer

Rectal cancer may have a greater direct effect on physical components of sexual functioning. Colon cancer is less likely to require radiotherapy and a permanent stoma. Comparisons of treatment modalities suggest a greater impact of radiotherapy, particularly preoperative radiotherapy, worsening sexual outcomes with an impact on secondary urinary symptoms. New nerve-sparing surgery has not been shown to be of benefit yet. Treatments including surgery, stomas, chemoradiotherapy or chemotherapy alone worsen overall quality of life and sexuality, with an individual response depending on age, gender and staging. Bowel dysfunction and poor stoma management increase sexual dysfunction with the stoma having the greatest impact, hopefully improving after and if the stoma is reversed. However, it is reported there was no difference in sexual function in women with rectal or colon cancer when radiotherapy was not used, but up to 50% did not resume sexual activity (64). Laparoscopic resection or sphincter-preserving surgery is better than an abdominoperineal resection/Hartman's for low rectal cancer with respect to body image and urinary symptoms but no difference for female sexual function or oncological risk (65).

Breast Cancer

Breast cancer survivors have the most data regarding body image, sexual functioning and sexuality. Women with early-stage breast cancer are twice as likely as the general population to suffer depression, which, coupled with anxiety, predicts QoL. The rates of sexual dysfunction are hugely variable (up to at least 75%) and may be influenced by the menopausal status of the individual. Perimenopausal complaints of poor sleep, low and labile mood, vasomotor symptoms and dyspareunia have consequences for sexual function domains of desire, arousal and orgasm, in addition to pain. Discussion of these factors is required at different stages of treatment and follow-up.

Treatments for Sexual Dysfunction

As has previously been discussed, sexual problems are common and even more prevalent in people diagnosed and treated with cancer. Discussing these issues and contextualising them for an individual can be a therapeutic intervention in itself. However some people may actively seek treatment for sexual problems—talking therapies, physical therapies and pharmaceutical treatment should be available via cancer services. Physiotherapy and sex therapists may provide additional support, but much counselling can be delivered by the core oncology team with a little additional training.

Hormonal Treatment

Hormonal effects of oestrogen and testosterone deficiency have a direct and indirect impact on sexual functioning. For some hormone receptor-sensitive cancers, hormone therapy may be contraindicated—this is covered in other chapters. Local hormonal treatment may be acceptable with minimal if any additional recurrence risk compared with systemic treatment—with significant benefit for QoL. Vaginal dryness and pathological discharge causing dyspareunia are significant contributors to survivor morbidity.

Both tamoxifen and aromatase inhibitors can have a direct detrimental effect on areas of sexual functioning in addition to the impact on menopausal symptoms that may impact the acceptability of these agents. Management needs to be carefully discussed. Neglect of these difficulties with resultant loss of libido and partner problems related to performance anxiety can be more difficult to address after delay.

Local Treatments

Local urogenital treatments include non-hormonal moisturisers which should be trialled prior to consideration of vaginal oestrogens for most hormone-sensitive tumours (see previous chapters). The use of a water-based non-hormonal moisturiser was reported to reduce dyspareunia and dryness by 60% compared with only 40% in a group of women with breast cancer (66). Moisturisers are not equivalent to lubricants which facilitate penetration, but do not generally improve the intrinsic tissue integrity. Multiple lubricant brands are available commercially, but globally available products such as vegetable and nut oils may also be helpful.

Vaginal oestrogens are available in pessary, cream, ring and ovule forms, each with different attributes for vulval, vaginal and bladder tissues, improving bladder overactivity, UTI, dyspareunia with subsequent impact on QoL and sexual functioning. The WHI writing group reported no increased risk of breast or uterine cancer or cardiovascular disease associated with using vaginal oestrogen (67), supported by a Finnish registry of over 18,000 women reporting no increased risk associated with vaginal oestrogens in the general population (68). Although an increase in oestradiol level has been detected systemically in women using aromatase inhibitors during the initial two-week loading dose, there has been no increase in breast cancer, but this is observational data. The risk of local oestrogens is lower for those using tamoxifen due to its selective (o)estrogen receptor modulator action (SERM) (69). Overall the balance of benefit and risk needs to be discussed after a trial of non-hormonal remoisturisers and/lubricants.

There has been much interest in testosterone and dehydroepiandrosterone (DHEA) as alternative sex steroid hormones, but they are aromatised to oestrogens, predominantly in fat but also at a local level (70). Data for a local DHEA product, prasterone, licensed for GSM management do not exist yet for its safety long term. The six-month VIBRA study investigating prasterone in women with breast cancer on aromatase inhibitors indicated encouraging results with no increase in oestradiol levels and an improvement in vaginal and sexual health (71). There are currently no commercially available local testosterone products in the UK. Systemic testosterone and oestrogen are discussed in other chapters—both having a role in sexual wellbeing and QoL.

Another oral SERM, ospemifene, has a license to treat GSM but not enough safety data to warrant routine prescribing to those with hormone-sensitive tumours but is an option for those with other cancers and GSM, not wanting to use a vaginal product.

Laser treatment for GSM is a more innovative treatment although not widely available in the UK in the NHS. It has been suggested to have a yet undefined role in management of GSM in postmenopausal women (72) but initial studies in breast cancer show no advantage over sham treatment (73).

There is some evidence for reduction in superficial pain using topical local anaesthetic prior to intercourse—from 88% to 33% (74).

Dilator Therapy

The use of dilators has been reviewed in a Cochrane database (75) to prevent stenosis after radiotherapy, with very rare side effects, although it should be limited during the acute phase of treatment.

For those receiving radiotherapy, at three years post diagnosis: 50% with endometrial cancer, 60% with cervical cancer and 80% with anal carcinoma had vaginal stenosis. Chemoradiotherapy, more commonly used for younger women with cervical cancer, can have an additionally toxic effect. Current lack of research has made it unclear who should train patients in their use, the timing relative to treatment in addition to frequency and duration. A recent review (76) has confirmed that education coupled with pelvic floor physiotherapy (multimodal treatment) benefits overall pelvic and sexual function for gynaecological cancers.

Decreased sensation or difficulty with penetration can be related to superficial dyspareunia due to atrophic changes, compounded by vaginal muscle spasm/vaginismus. Although both can be related, with the bodily reaction to pain causing vaginismus, it is important to differentiate between the two because the modality of treatment may be different. This requires physical assessment by trained practitioners. Treatment often recommended is vaginal dilator, or more correctly, trainer therapy which is believed to be helpful for vaginismus—this may be supported or unsupported. Fingers or sex toys may be more useful to de-medicalise, and sex play may be more helpful to reengage with a sense of sexual self, with or without a partner. Dilators, manual therapy and biofeedback can be helpful for those with vaginal stenosis after radiotherapy or due to vulvovaginal atrophy secondary to oestrogen deficiency.

Vaginal dilation may be appropriate for most patients, irrespective of their partner status, although those with partners continuing sexual activity may maintain vaginal patency. Support can be delivered by the oncology team—doctors and nurses, a psychosexual counsellor (although they may not examine patients and therefore have limited understanding of the physical restrictions) and/or physiotherapists. Interestingly one study indicated dilator use after brachytherapy did not improve vaginal dimensions, but compared to controls had reduced constipation, dryness and urinary incontinence (77).

Sex Therapy

Loss of desire will be dependent on pre-diagnosis functioning, but post treatment, psychosexual counselling, cognitive behavioural therapy, sensate focus (a structured programme for reengaging with sexual activity), PLISSIT (permission, limited information, specific suggestions, intensive therapy) model and hypnosis are all options for survivor support. However, the cancer support team may also help by reviewing the impact of hormone blockers, such as tamoxifen and aromatase inhibitors, use of antidepressants and other treatment induced conditions including oestrogen deficiency.

Nonhormonal Medication

There has been much interest in medications for hypoactive sexual desire disorder (loss of arousal and desire). Flibanserin is licensed in the US but has significant side effects and interactions with alcohol, and requires daily dosing (78). The injectable bremelanotide, a melanocortin receptor agonist, has data proving its benefit in premenopausal women with loss of desire and concomitant distress (79) but no studies in a cancer population. Bupropion, a dopaminergic agent, had data to suggest it was beneficial for cancer-induced sexual dysfunction (low desire being licensed use in the US) but subsequent studies have not confirmed this (80).

See further Boxes 6.1 and 6.2.

BOX 6.1   TREATMENTS FOR SEXUAL DYSFUNCTION AFTER CANCER

Psychological support pre and post diagnosis
Psychosexual counselling
Dilator use
Management of oestrogen deficiency—local and systemic
Local treatment—vaginal moisturisers and lubricants
Systemic treatments
Physiotherapy: pelvic floor/musculoskeletal

BOX 6.2   HOW TO HELP PREVENT AND TREAT SEXUAL DYSFUNCTION

Addressing sexual issues at every and any opportunity
Permission giving
Timing of discussions—more emphasis post treatment
Written/online information to consolidate individual conversations
Decision making aids for treatment pathways
Basic training for all healthcare professionals
Referral pathway to psychosexual specialist and/or psychological support
Timely basic advice regarding simple interventions

LGBTQI/LGBTQ+

More inclusive healthcare for the LGBTQI+ community is imperative for improving the quality of care and negative impact of perceived discrimination. Healthcare systems can be problematic with recording sensitive information regarding sexual orientation and gender. This is even more marked for the trans population, binary and non-binary. The difficulties amongst healthcare professionals in asking about sexual orientation and gender identity present significant issues for trans people negotiating cancer care that may vary with the cis LGBQ population. Screening programmes are less readily undertaken (or less consistently invited for) by the trans population which may be related to an increase in cancer compared with the cis population (81). This includes cervical screening for trans men and prostate screening amongst trans women. Although some studies have suggested exogenous gender affirmation hormone therapy increases cancer incidence, the evidence for this is low but requires further research (82).

Cancer interventions may disrupt gender affirmation interventions and increase gender dysphoria. However, the converse may be true that treatments such as mastectomy may contribute to gender euphoria. There is increasing evidence for people with a cancer diagnosis accelerating their decisions regarding gender affirmation (83).

Training of healthcare professionals in trans care and those cis individuals who are gay, lesbian or queer, with improvement in healthcare systems and data management, will facilitate respectful interactions with healthcare institutions and improve care for all people with a cancer diagnosis.

Conclusion

Recovery of sexual health and intimate relationships is a frequently undervalued component of quality of life and wellbeing, both by healthcare professionals and patients. Lesser engagement with the consequences of the cancer journey with women may be due to the perceived limitations of treatment for female sexual dysfunction. However with some training, the multiprofessional team can manage these aspects of care. This will allow for greater individualisation of management, incorporating both patient wishes and the available appropriate data. This may require a variety of approaches with different HCPs. It has been proven that this is appreciated by patients and their partners, facilitating shared decision making. Multimodal treatment should be available to those who need it—physiotherapists, sex therapists, fertility specialists, hormone experts etc.

A therapeutic approach tailored not just to pathology but to the individual patient, delivered by good communication within a multidisciplinary team, will do much to address issues regarding sexuality, body image and fertility.

References

1. National Institute of Cancer. Cancer Statistics [internet], 2024. Available from: www.cancer.gov/about-cancer/understanding/statistics.
2. MacMillan Support. Cancer Sstatistics in the UK [internet]. Available from: www.macmillan.org.uk/about-us/what-we-do/research/cancer-statistics-fact-sheet#:~:text=New%20cases%20of%20cancer%20diagnosed,at%20least%20every%2090%20seconds.&text=Due%20to%20the%20disruption%20caused,12%25%20between%202019%20and%202020.
3. Cancer Research UK. Cancer Incidence for Common Cancers [internet], 2024. Available from: www.cancerresearchuk.org/health-professional/cancer-statistics/incidence/common-cancers-compared#:~:text=Breast%20cancer%20is%20the%20most%20common%20cancer%20in%20UK%20females,and%20bowel%20cancer%20(11%25).
4. WHO. Sexual Health [internet], 2024. Available from: www.who.int/health-topics/sexual-health#tab=tab_1.
5. McCool ME et al. Prevalence of female sexual dysfunction among premenopausal women: A systematic review and meta-analysis of observational studies. Sex Med Rev. 2016;4(3):197–212.
6. Plouffe L Jr. Screening for sexual problems through a simple questionnaire. Am J Obstet Gynecol. 1985;151(2):166–9.
7. Sikorska M et al. The impact of HPV Diagnosis and the Electrosurgical Excision Procedure (LEEP) on mental health and sexual functioning: A systematic review. Cancers (Basel). 2023;15(8).
8. Clayton AH et al. The Changes in Sexual Functioning Questionnaire (CSFQ): Development, reliability, and validity. Psychopharmacol Bull. 1997;33(4):731–45.
9. Rosen R et al. The Female Sexual Function Index (FSFI): A multidimensional self-report instrument for the assessment of female sexual function. J Sex Marital Ther. 2000;26(2):191–208.
10. European Organisation for Research and Treatment of Cancer. Available from: www.eortc.org/.
11. Jeffery DD et al. Self-reported sexual function measures administered to female cancer patients: A systematic review, 2008–2014. J Psychosoc Oncol. 2015;33(4):433–66.
12. Flynn KE et al. Patient experiences with communication about sex during and after treatment for cancer. Psychooncol. 2012;21(6):594–601.
13. Taylor J et al. Sexual health toxicity in cancer survivors: Is there a gender disparity in physician evaluation and intervention? Int J Radiation Oncol Biol Phys. 2020;108(3):S136.
14. Institute of Psychosexual Medicine. Available from: www.ipm.org.uk.
15. Zangeneh S et al. A silence full of words: Sociocultural beliefs behind the sexual health of Iranian women undergoing breast cancer treatment, a qualitative study. Support Care Cancer. 2022;31(1):84.

16. Lindau ST et al. A manifesto on the preservation of sexual function in women and girls with cancer. Am J Obstet Gynecol. 2015;213(2):166–74.

17. Stein KD et al. Physical and psychological long-term and late effects of cancer. Cancer. 2008;112(11_suppl):2577–92.

18. Webber L et al. ESHRE guideline: Management of women with premature ovarian insufficiency. Hum Reprod. 2016;31(5):926–37.

19. Dunlop CE, Anderson RA. Uses of Anti-Müllerian Hormone (AMH) measurement before and after cancer treatment in women. Maturitas. 2015;80(3):245–50.

20. WHO. WHOQOL: Measuring Quality of Life [internet], 2012. Available from: www.who.int/tools/whoqol.

21. Wilmoth MC, Spinelli A. Sexual implications of gynecologic cancer treatments. J Obstet Gynecol Neonatal Nurs. 2000;29(4):413–21.

22. Shisler R et al. Life after endometrial cancer: A systematic review of patient-reported outcomes. Gynecol Oncol. 2018;148(2):403–13.

23. Logue CA et al. Psychosexual morbidity in women with ovarian cancer. Int J Gynecol Cancer. 2020;30(12):1983–9.

24. Palaia I et al. Long-term quality of life and sexual function after neoadjuvant chemotherapy and radical surgery for locally advanced cervical cancer. J Sex Med. 2022;19(4):613–19.

25. Ramirez PT et al. Minimally invasive versus abdominal radical hysterectomy for cervical cancer. N Engl J Med. 2018;379(20):1895–904.

26. Uccella S et al. Sexual function following laparoscopic versus transvaginal closure of the vaginal vault after laparoscopic hysterectomy: Secondary analysis of a randomized trial by the Italian society of gynecological endoscopy using a validated questionnaire. J Minim Invas Gynecol. 2020;27(1):186–94.

27. Gueli Alletti S et al. Single-institution propensity-matched study to evaluate the psychological effect of minimally invasive interval debulking surgery versus standard laparotomic treatment: From body to mind and back. J Minim Invasive Gynecol. 2018;25(5):816–22.

28. Membrilla-Beltran L et al. Impact of cervical cancer on quality of life and sexuality in female survivors. Int J Environ Res Public Health. 2023;20(4).

29. White ID et al. Assessment of treatment-induced female sexual morbidity in oncology: Is this a part of routine medical follow-up after radical pelvic radiotherapy? Br J Cancer. 2011;105(7):903–10.

30. Fingeret MC et al. Managing body image difficulties of adult cancer patients: Lessons from available research. Cancer. 2014;120(5):633–41.

31. Verri V et al. The influence of body image on psychological symptomatology in breast cancer women undergoing intervention: A pre-post study. Front Psychol. 2024;15.

32. James W. The Principles of Psychology. New York: Henry Holt; 1890.

33. Pitcher S et al. Holistic sexuality post gynaecological cancer treatment: A review of recent literature. South African J Oncol. 2018;2.

34. National Institute of Cancer. Body Image [internet], 2024. Available from: www.cancer.gov/publications/dictionaries/cancer-terms/def/body-image.

35. Cash TF. Cognitive-behavioral perspectives on body image. In: Cash T, ed. Encyclopedia of Body Image and Human Appearance. Oxford: Academic Press; 2012: 334–42.

36. Fredrickson BL, Roberts T-A. Objectification theory: Toward understanding women's lived experiences and mental health risks. Psychol Women Q. 1997;21(2):173–206.

37. White CA. Body image dimensions and cancer: A heuristic cognitive behavioural model. Psychooncol. 2000;9(3):183–92.

38. Kleinman A. Culture and Depression: Studies in the Antropology and Cross-Cultural Psychiatry of Affect and Disorder. Los Angeles: University of California Press; 1985.

39. Fobair P et al. Body image and sexual problems in young women with breast cancer. Psychooncol. 2006;15(7):579–94.

40. Sacerdoti RC et al. Altered sexuality and body image after gynecological cancer treatment: How can psychologists help? Prof Psychol Res Pract. 2010;41(6):533–40.

41. Solbrække KN, Bondevik H. Absent organs—present selves: Exploring embodiment and gender iden- tity in young Norwegian women's accounts of hysterectomy. Int J Qual Stud Health Well-being. 2015;10:26720.

42. Teo I et al. The relationship between symptom prevalence, body image, and quality of life in Asian gynecologic cancer patients. Psychooncol. 2018;27(1):69–74.

43. Wilson CM et al. Body image, sexuality, and sexual functioning in women with gynecologic cancer: An integrative review of the literature and implications for research. Cancer Nurs. 2021;44(5):E252–86.

44. Krouse R et al. Quality of life outcomes in 599 cancer and non-cancer patients with colostomies. J Surg Res. 2007;138(1):79–87.

45. Zhu X et al. Sexual experiences of Chinese patients living with an ostomy. J Wound Ostomy Cont Nurs. 2017;44(5):469–74.

46. Deshpande PS, Gupta AS. Causes and prevalence of factors causing infertility in a public health facil- ity. J Hum Reprod Sci. 2019;12(4):287–93.

47. Benedict C et al. Fertility issues in adolescent and young adult cancer survivors. J Adolesc Young Adult Oncol. 2016;5(1):48–57.

48. Karen KW et al. Cancer as a "we-disease": Examining the process of coping from a relational perspec- tive. Fam Syst Health. 2007;25(4):404–18.

49. Manne S, Badr H. Intimacy and relationship processes in couples' psychosocial adaptation to cancer. Cancer. 2008;112(11_suppl):2541–55.

50. Hawkey A et al. Talking but not always understanding: Couple communication about infertility concerns after cancer. BMC Public Health. 2021;21(1):161.

51. Reulen RC et al. Pregnancy and labor complications in female survivors of childhood cancer: The British Childhood Cancer Survivor Study. J Natl Cancer Inst. 2017;109(11).

52. Teh WT et al. The impact of uterine radiation on subsequent fertility and pregnancy outcomes. Biomed Res. Int. 2014;2014(1):482968.

53. van den Berg M et al. Development and testing of a tailored online fertility preservation decision aid for female cancer patients. Cancer Med. 2021;10(5):1576–88.

54. Bennett KF et al. The psychosexual impact of testing positive for high-risk cervical human papilloma- virus (HPV): A systematic review. Psychooncol. 2019;28(10):1959–70.

55. Drolet M et al. Population-level impact and herd effects following the introduction of human papillomavirus vaccination programmes: Updated systematic review and meta-analysis. Lancet. 2019;394(10197):497–509.

56. Chrysostomou AC et al. Cervical cancer screening programs in Europe: The transition towards HPV vaccination and population-based HPV testing. Viruses. 2018;10(12).

57. Flay LD, Matthews JH. The effects of radiotherapy and surgery on the sexual function of women treated for cervical cancer. Int J Radiat Oncol Biol Phys. 1995;31(2):399–404.

58. Bergmark K et al. Vaginal changes and sexuality in women with a history of cervical cancer. N Engl J Med. 1999;340(18):1383–9.

59. Cianci S et al. Post treatment sexual function and quality of life of patients affected by cervical cancer: A systematic review. Medicina (Kaunas). 2023;59(4).

60. Tsatsou I et al. A systematic review of sexuality and depression of cervical cancer patients. J Sex Marital Ther. 2019;45(8):739–54.

61. Warring S et al. The quality of life after endometrial cancer study: Baseline characteristics and patient- reported outcomes. Curr Oncol. 2024;31(9):5557–72.

62. Malandrone F et al. The impact of vulvar cancer on psychosocial and sexual functioning: A literature review. Cancers. 2021;14(1).

63. Martin R et al. Female sexual function in bladder cancer: A review of the evidence. BJUI Compass. 2023;4(1):5–23.

64. Thyø A et al. Female sexual problems after treatment for colorectal cancer—a population-based study. Colorectal Dis. 2019;21(10):1130–9.

65. Kang SB et al. Quality of life after sphincter preservation surgery or abdominoperineal resection for low rectal cancer (ASPIRE): A long-term prospective, multicentre, cohort study. Lancet Reg Health West Pac. 2021;6:100087.

66. Loprinzi CL et al. Phase III randomized double-blind study to evaluate the efficacy of a polycarbo-phil-based vaginal moisturizer in women with breast cancer. J Clin Oncol. 1997;15(3):969–73.
67. Crandall CJ et al. Breast cancer, endometrial cancer, and cardiovascular events in participants who used vaginal estrogen in the Women's Health Initiative Observational Study. Menopause. 2018;25(1):11–20.
68. Lyytinen H et al. Breast cancer risk in postmenopausal women using estrogen-only therapy. Obstet Gynecol. 2006;108(6):1354–60.
69. Le Ray I et al. Local estrogen therapy and risk of breast cancer recurrence among hormone-treated patients: A nested case-control study. Breast Cancer Res Treat. 2012;135(2):603–9.
70. Hussain I, Talaulikar VS. A systematic review of randomised clinical trials—the safety of vaginal hormones and selective estrogen receptor modulators for the treatment of genitourinary menopausal symptoms in breast cancer survivors. Post Reprod Health. 2023;29(4):222–31.
71. Mension E et al. Safety of prasterone in breast cancer survivors treated with aromatase inhibitors: The VIBRA pilot study. Climacteric. 2022;25(5):476–82.
72. Liu M et al. Efficacy of CO_2 laser treatment in postmenopausal women with vulvovaginal atrophy: A meta-analysis. Int J Gynaecol Obstet. 2022;158(2):241–51.
73. Mension E et al. Effect of fractional carbon dioxide vs sham laser on sexual function in survivors of breast cancer receiving aromatase inhibitors for genitourinary syndrome of menopause: The LIGHT randomized clinical trial. JAMA Netw Open. 2023;6(2):e2255697.
74. Goetsch MF et al. A practical solution for dyspareunia in breast cancer survivors: A randomized controlled trial. J Clin Oncol. 2015;33(30):3394–400.
75. Miles T, Johnson N. Vaginal dilator therapy for women receiving pelvic radiotherapy. Cochrane Database Syst Rev. 2014;2014(9):Cd007291.
76. Cyr MP et al. Effectiveness of pelvic floor muscle and education-based therapies on bladder, bowel, vaginal, sexual, psychological function, quality of life, and pelvic floor muscle function in females treated for gynecological cancer: A systematic review. Curr Oncol Rep. 2024;26(11):1293–320.
77. Cerentini TM et al. Clinical and psychological outcomes of the use of vaginal dilators after gynaecological brachytherapy: A randomized clinical trial. Adv Ther. 2019;36(8):1936–49.
78. Katz M et al. Efficacy of flibanserin in women with hypoactive sexual desire disorder: Results from the BEGONIA trial. J Sex Med. 2013;10(7):1807–15.
79. Kingsberg SA et al. Bremelanotide for the treatment of hypoactive sexual desire disorder: Two randomized phase 3 trials. Obstet Gynecol. 2019;134(5):899–908.
80. Barton DL et al. Randomized controlled phase II evaluation of two dose levels of bupropion versus placebo for sexual desire in female cancer survivors: NRG-CC004. J Clin Oncol. 2022;40(4):324–34.
81. Peitzmeier SM et al. Enacting power and constructing gender in cervical cancer screening encounters between transmasculine patients and health care providers. Cult Health Sex. 2020;22(12):1315–32.
82. Jackson SS, Hammer A. Cancer risk among transgender adults: A growing population with unmet needs. Acta Obstet Gynecol Scand. 2023;102(11):1428–30.
83. Ussher JM et al. Reinforcing or disrupting gender affirmation: The impact of cancer on transgender embodiment and identity. Arch Sex Behav. 2023;52(3):901–20.

Chapter 7

Female Fertility Assessment and Preservation Procedures for Cancer Survivors

Elizabeth Varghese, Kirsten Das and Jacqueline C. Yano Maher

Epidemiology and Impact of Chemotherapy and Radiation on the Female Reproductive System

In the United States, there are currently approximately 400,000 female cancer survivors who are of childbearing age (1, 2). The most frequent cancer types in children and adolescents include leukemia, lymphoma, neuroblastoma, and sarcoma. Given significant treatment advancements, many of these cancers are now treatable. In developed countries, the five-year survival rate for childhood cancers is over 80% (3). Furthermore, there is a rising trend in early-onset cancers in female patients under the age of 50, potentially increasing the population of females of childbearing age undergoing treatment (4).

Chemotherapy affects the ovaries as it targets the rapidly dividing granulosa cells and oocytes. This then leads to the destruction of growing ovarian follicles. Certain chemotherapy drugs, including alkylating agents, platinum compounds, and anthracycline antibiotics, are particularly harmful to the ovaries by damaging DNA strands and generating excessive reactive oxygen species (5), which accelerates the activation, inflammation, and apoptosis of primordial follicles (6). These treatments also harm ovarian blood vessels leading to fibrosis of the ovarian cortex, further decreasing the survival of primordial follicles (7, 8).

Like chemotherapy, radiation treatment also leads to the loss of oocytes and granulosa cells, reduced ovarian follicle count, vascular damage, and increased stromal fibrosis. Radiation type, dose, and duration impact ovarian reserve and rates of premature ovarian insufficiency (POI) with younger patients less affected (9). According to the "Fertility Risk Calculator" from the University of Pittsburgh, whole abdominal and pelvic radiation doses of >10 Gy in postpubertal girls and >15 Gy in prepubertal girls is associated with a significant risk of gonadotoxicity leading to infertility (10). Prepubertal patients typically have a better chance of preserving fertility, largely due to a greater ovarian reserve at treatment initiation (11) and the ovaries being in a quiescent

DOI: 10.1201/9781032631028-7

state. Radiation can also impact the uterus, which can lead to difficulty conceiving, increased rates of miscarriage, placental insufficiency, premature birth, low birth weight, perinatal death, and poor obstetrical outcomes (12–15). Uterine radiation is estimated to cause uterine dysfunction between 14–30 Gy (16–18). However, even doses as low as 4 Gy have been shown to have an effect on fertility (15), with prepubertal uteri more prone to injury than adult women with a uterus that has finished growing (12, 19).

There are well-established female fertility preservation guidelines prior to undergoing cancer treatment from the American Society of Reproductive Medicine (ASRM) (20), the American Society of Clinical Oncology (ASCO) (21), and the European Society of Human Reproduction and Embryology (ESHRE) (22). However, there remains a need for comprehensive fertility preservation and reproductive health guidelines for cancer survivors post treatment, particularly among those who were children, adolescents, and young adults at the time of diagnosis (23).

Fertility Preservation before Cancer Treatment

The 2019 ASRM recommendations emphasize the importance of early and informed decision-making to preserve reproductive potential of young cancer patients (20). There are a variety of options that vary in efficacy including 1) oocyte/embryo cryopreservation ("egg" or embryo freezing), 2) ovarian tissue cryopreservation (OTC), removing ovarian tissue and re-transplanting it at a later time, 3) use of gonadotropin-releasing hormone (GnRH) agonists, and 4) ovarian or 5) uterine transposition, surgically moving the ovary or uterus from the pelvis to avoid radiation (20).

Oocyte/Embryo Cryopreservation

Embryo and oocyte cryopreservation is the standard of care for fertility preservation. Embryo cryopreservation is a fertility preservation method whereby fertilized embryos (typically day 5–6 blastocysts) are frozen, which is particularly beneficial for individuals or couples who have viable sperm and oocytes prior to treatment. In younger patients, its use may involve more complex ethical and legal considerations (24). Oocyte cryopreservation involves freezing unfertilized oocytes, offering an option for those without a current partner or who prefer not to use donor sperm. ASRM lifted the experimental label from oocyte cryopreservation in 2012 (25). Both techniques are typically available only to post-menarchal patients.

Chemotherapy can significantly reduce oocyte quantity and possibly quality (26–28). Additionally, embryo and oocyte cryopreservation often require a minimum of 10–14 days for controlled ovarian stimulation (COS) and an additional one to two weeks to obtain an appointment at a fertility center and medical care coordination (29). A GnRH antagonist protocol is often used to stimulate the ovarian follicles, which includes gonadotropins followed by the addition of a GnRH antagonist to prevent premature ovulation. For patients with estrogen-sensitive cancers such as breast cancer, an aromatase inhibitor (letrozole) 5 mg daily can be added starting on the first day of stimulation and continuing to 7 days after the oocyte retrieval (30). A trigger shot of human chorionic gonadotropin (hCG) or GnRH agonists allows for the final maturation step prior to oocyte retrieval (29, 31). Random start and conventional start ovarian stimulation have shown similar mature oocyte yield (32).

During COS, the progression of follicle development is observed via pelvic ultrasound (usually abdominal in children/adolescents, transvaginal in older adolescents/adults) and serum hormone testing. Oocyte retrieval is performed by an ultrasound-guided transvaginal needle aspiration under anesthesia. The harvested oocytes are then removed from surrounding cumulus cells, and the fully mature oocytes (metaphase II) are cryopreserved. If cryopreserving embryos, the mature oocytes undergo fertilization using either conventional in-vitro fertilization (IVF), which involves incubating the oocytes with sperm, or through intracytoplasmic sperm injection (ICSI), whereby the sperm is directly injected into the oocyte (31, 33). Following fertilization, embryos are cultured to the blastocyst stage (approximately five or six days) and then undergo cryopreservation (34). In the past, oocytes and embryos were typically cryopreserved using a slow-freezing method (35, 36). The preferred technique now is vitrification, a quick cooling process that considerably minimizes the formation of ice crystals in cells and is more time-efficient (37).

Historically, embryos cryopreserve better than oocytes because mature oocytes are more susceptible to damage given their larger size, higher water content, lower surface-to-volume ratio, and presence of meiotic spindles (38, 39). These spindles are prone to temperature-induced damage, potentially causing chromosomal irregularities post fertilization (40). The older slow-freezing method frequently led to the formation of ice crystals, thereby reducing the success rates of oocyte preservation. However, advancements in vitrification have significantly enhanced outcomes, demonstrating high survival rates of oocytes post thaw, along with successful fertilization and pregnancy rates that are on par with those of fresh embryos and oocytes (41). In 2017, Ho et al. did not find significant differences in clinical pregnancy outcomes, rates of live births, or perinatal results between the use of thawed oocytes and embryos that were cryopreserved (42).

When looking at the safety of COS in the AYA population, a study by Manuel et al. performed a sub-analysis on their cancer patients ages 13–21. Out of 41 patients, 38 were successfully stimulated, had mature oocytes retrieved and cryopreserved, and had no adverse events. Data showed that when comparing patients ages 13–17 to patients 18–21 years, there was no statistical difference in total dose of gonadotropins, number of days stimulated, or number of mature oocytes retrieved. The median number of oocytes cryopreserved were 11 and 13, respectively (43).

Ovarian Tissue Cryopreservation

Ovarian tissue cryopreservation (OTC) and transplantation (OTT) are processes in which ovarian tissue is removed surgically, typically prior to cancer treatment, and re-implanted surgically back into the body when a patient is ready for pregnancy. It has gained recognition as a standard fertility preservation method for patients undergoing gonadotoxic treatments and is no longer considered experimental per ASRM as of 2019 (20, 44). OTC is currently the standard of care for prepubertal girls and an option for postpubertal girls and women who cannot delay cancer treatment to cryopreserve oocytes/embryos. OTC followed by OTT has resulted in over 200 live births (45) and also has been shown to restore reproductive endocrine function (20). Potential risks include the possible reintroduction of malignant cells, especially in leukemia patients, as well as limitations in long-term pregnancy data in niche populations (46, 47).

In this technique, a part of or the entire ovary is extracted via minimally invasive laparoscopic surgery. The surgical technique varies by fertility preservation center and surgeon experience, and the amount of tissue removed has varied from multiple cortical biopsies, partial oophorectomy, or complete unilateral oophorectomy (48). At the authors' institutions it is preferred to perform a unilateral oophorectomy (laparoscopic approach unless an open resection or debulking is performed by general surgery) and utilize cold scissors and blunt dissection for removal whenever possible to minimize thermal spread and damage to the ovary and its follicles. Preference is for right ovary removal over left because 1) the lack of sigmoid colon in the right pelvis oftentimes makes it easier to dissect and remove the right ovary, 2) there is increased risk of right-sided ovarian torsion in the general population, and 3) the appendix is located on the right, thus removing the right ovary will make the differential diagnosis of right lower quadrant pain easier in the future. However, the left ovary can be removed if the right ovary is surgically more challenging, will endure more radiation, or is compromised by another clinical factor. Suggested surgical steps for the laparoscopic procedure are as follows. The utero-ovarian ligament is identified and grasped with a Maryland grasper. Sharp laparoscopic scissors are then utilized to take down the mesosalpinx. Care is taken to separate the fallopian tube away from the ovary. Given pubertal status and blood supply, monopolar laparoscopic scissors or a vessel sealing device, preferably a harmonic scalpel, is utilized. Once the infundibular pelvic (IP) ligament is skeletonized, an endoscopic ligating loop (e.g. Endo Loop) is used to suture ligate the gonadal blood vessels supplying the ovary. The IP ligament is then cut with laparoscopic scissors and the ovary is removed from pelvis (49). If the IP is large or the pedicle is thick, a vessel sealing device can be used to ligate the IP instead. The ovary is then immediately placed in tissue holding media and processed in an embryology laboratory as soon as possible. For best cryopreservation, it is recommended that the ovarian medulla is removed until a thickness of 1–1.5 mm of ovarian cortex remains, since this is where the primordial follicles reside (50). The cortex is then sliced into strips and cryopreserved. More recently vitrification of ovarian tissue has been attempted successfully (51); however, slow freezing has been utilized longer, shown better outcomes in terms of tissue survival, and currently has more live births reported (27).

When patients are ready to have children, strips of cryopreserved ovarian tissue are autologously transplanted back into the patient through OTT. The transplanted ovarian cortical fragments are typically placed back into the pelvic or peritoneal cavity (orthotopic sites), but attempts have also been made to graft them in non-traditional locations like the forearm or anterior abdominal wall (heterotopic sites). Common transplantation sites include the remaining non-functional ovary or the peritoneal bursa (52).

For postpubertal patients, combining OTC with oocyte/embryo freezing presents an innovative approach to enhance fertility preservation. OTC can be timed before, during, or after COS depending on various factors, including time, ovarian response to stimulation, and cancer treatment status (53, 54). Studies indicate that tissue harvesting does not impact the quantity or quality of mature oocytes retrieved post COS (55).

GnRH Agonists

GnRH agonists given in a sustained fashion such as a one-month or three-month Depo intramuscular injection, after an initial surge, suppresses gonadotropin release of follicle-stimulating hormone (FSH) and luteinizing hormone (LH) and thus downregulates the hypothalamic-pituitary-ovarian (HPO) axis (56). The POEMS (Prevention of Early Menopause Study) trial, involving 257 breast cancer patients, revealed that GnRHa have some protection against POI during chemotherapy and improve pregnancy rates (57). Despite their promise in breast cancer patients, the effectiveness of GnRH agonists in other populations for fertility preservation remains under investigation.

Limited data exists over the efficacy of GnRH agonists for fertility preservation in cancer patients. Several studies did not show a significant increase in cumulative ovarian function with GnRHa (58). Specifically, initial studies by Demeestere et al. found no difference in POI rates between GnRHa and control groups after one year of follow-up, but two years of follow-up then indicated better ovarian function restoration and higher anti-Mullerian hormone (AMH) levels in the GnRHa group (59, 60). Ultimately, GnRH agonists can be offered as an adjunct to embryo, oocyte, and tissue cryopreservation options, especially to manage or prevent heavy menstrual bleeding during cancer treatment, but should not serve as a replacement (61).

Ovarian Transposition

Ovarian transposition is a surgical procedure used in fertility preservation for patients undergoing pelvic radiation. It involves repositioning the ovaries out of the radiation field, usually higher in the abdomen, to protect them from radiation-induced damage (62). It is sometimes used with gynecological cancers, sarcomas, or Hodgkin's lymphoma. One study noted an 88.6% success rate in preserving ovarian function (63). However, limitations include potential incidental radiation, ovarian cyst formation, and the need for additional fertility preservation methods (64, 65).

Uterine Transposition and Transplantation

The increasing number of young patients with tumors, particularly colorectal cancers, has necessitated innovative fertility preservation techniques. Pelvic radiation therapy, often part of the treatment for these cancers, can lead to infertility by affecting the ovaries and uterus. The technique of uterine transposition, initially introduced by Ribeiro et al. in 2017 for rectal cancer, offers a promising option for preserving reproductive function (66). It entails detaching the uterus from the vagina and temporarily moving the uterus along with the fallopian tubes and ovaries up towards the abdominal wall to safeguard the uterus against pelvic radiation. The cervix is then sutured to the paracolic gutter (if menses is suppressed) or to the umbilicus (to allow for menstrual bleeding) (67, 68). This method has been successfully applied in various cases, including a pediatric patient in 2021, and marked a significant achievement with the first successful live birth reported in 2023 following the procedure (69).

Gynecologic Cancers and Surgical Sparing Methods

There is a role for fertility-sparing surgical interventions in certain gynecologic cancers. If fertility is desired, early-stage cervical cancer can be treated with a cervical excisional procedure or a trachelectomy, both allowing for potential pregnancy in the future with definitive treatment after childbearing is complete (70). Additionally, endometrial hyperplasia and early-stage endometrial cancer have been treated by various fertility-sparing methods including oral progestins such as medroxyprogesterone acetate or megestrol acetate, levonorgestrel intrauterine devices, hysteroscopic resection, or a combination (71, 72). There is no consensus on choice of treatment or dosing. This can be considered for patients who have plans to conceive in the near future but requires close surveillance and should be individualized. Furthermore, some ovarian tumors in young adolescents, such as a dysgerminoma or borderline tumors, can be considered for conservative management with an ovarian cystectomy rather than oophorectomy (73, 74).

Ovarian Reserve Surveillance Post Treatment

A patient's ovarian reserve or total number of oocytes undergoes an anticipated decline starting from 16–20 weeks of gestation until menopause (75). At birth, there are approximately 1 to 2 million oocytes. However, by the time of puberty, this number has already decreased to 300,000–500,000 oocytes. By the age of 40, approximately 5% of oocytes remain from puberty, which translates to approximately 10,000 to 25,000, varying from person to person. At the time

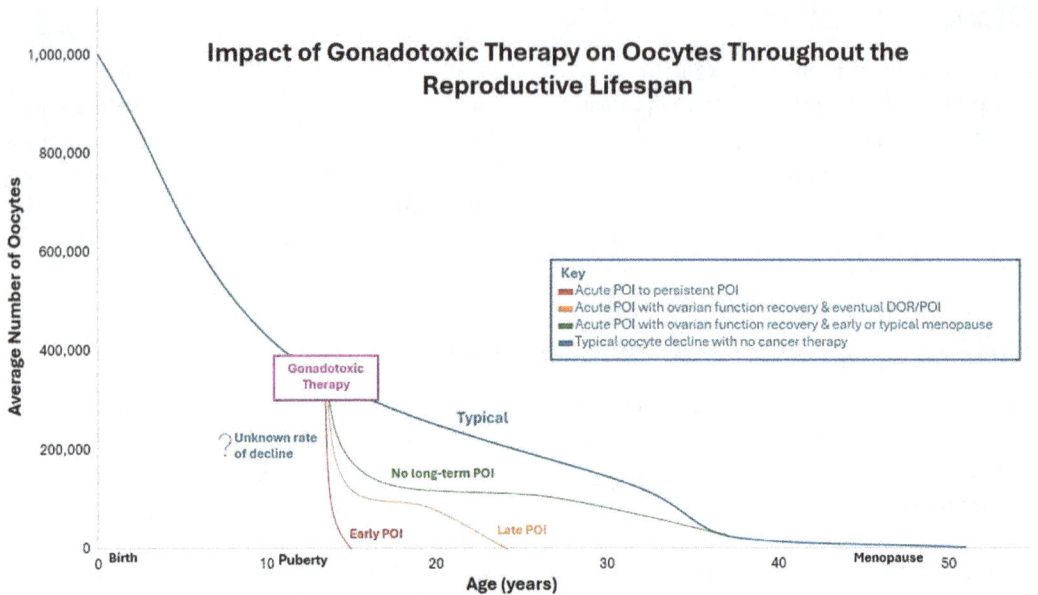

Figure 7.1 Schematic of the impact of gonadotoxic treatment on the number of oocytes throughout the reproductive lifespan.

of menopause, there are few (<1,000) remaining viable oocytes (76). Any remaining follicles are typically resistant to hormonal stimulation required for ovulation, marking the end of the natural reproductive lifespan. In addition to quantity of oocytes, quality and ability to conceive with those oocytes also decreases with age (77, 78). Figure 7.1 represents a schematic of the proposed impact gonadotoxic therapy has on oocyte number if treated during the adolescent years and three potential outcomes.

Launched in 1980, the Childhood Cancer Survivor Study (CCSS) aimed to monitor the long-term health outcomes of children who survived pediatric cancer (79). From 1970 to 1986, a CCSS cohort noted a reduced probability of pregnancy (RR 0.8) in female survivors compared to their non-affected siblings (80) and from 1970 to 1999, there was a lower pregnancy rate in survivors attempting to conceive over 30 years old (HR 0.6) (81). Furthermore, POI before the age of 40 occurred in 8% of survivors, compared to 0.8% in unaffected female siblings (82). There was a 6% chance of acute ovarian insufficiency following treatment with greater risk in patients (a) over 13 years old, (b) treated with alkylating chemotherapy, and (c) receiving higher doses of radiation to the ovaries (83). The CCSS provides strong evidence that childhood cancer survivors have a lower likelihood of achieving pregnancy and an elevated risk of developing POI compared to their siblings (84).

Ovarian Reserve Testing

Ovarian reserve describes the quantity and quality of a patient's remaining oocyte supply, which naturally decreases with age until the average of menopause at 51 years. It can be estimated and evaluated through various serum markers that can indicate diminishing ovarian reserve.

Follicle-stimulating hormone (FSH), anti-Mullerian hormone (AMH), and antral follicle count (AFC) using transvaginal ultrasound are commonly used to assess ovarian reserve, providing insights into ovarian function and egg supply.

Prepubertal

Prepubertal girls can tolerate higher doses of alkylating agent chemotherapy and have a more preserved ovarian reserve (103), possibly because they have a great follicular pool of oocytes at the time of cancer treatment and/or the ovary is quiescent since follicles are not growing. For survivors who have not yet started or completed puberty, it is important to monitor their growth and sexual development (Sexual Maturity Rating or Tanner stage) annually post cancer treatment to identify abnormal puberty development and possible development of POI.

The Children's Oncology Group (COG) advises yearly evaluations that assess a patient's onset and tempo of puberty, menstrual history, sexual function, menopausal symptoms, medication use, and Tanner staging until sexually mature (105), as well as LH, FSH, and estradiol assessment when a patient reaches 13 years old (106). In clinical practice, the authors of this chapter believe it is reasonable to start evaluating girls over 11–12 years old with annual AMH, FSH, LH, and estradiol every one to two years after cancer treatment is complete to assess puberty, risk of acute ovarian failure, diminished ovarian reserve, and primary ovarian sufficiency. AMH values are less clear in prepubertal girls. If a patient exhibits no signs of puberty by age 13, or if pubertal development is not progressing as expected, further testing should be carried out (106), and pubertal induction or hormone replacement may be indicated.

FSH (Follicle-Stimulating Hormone)

When measured during the early follicular phase, on menstrual cycle days two through four, FSH is understood to reflect the basal or unregulated level of FSH due to ovarian feedback mechanisms to the pituitary gland (85). While day two through four FSH monitoring is not the sole method for evaluating ovarian reserve, it is a commonly acknowledged biomarker, offering a degree of reliability (86). The major limitation in utilizing FSH as a biomarker for ovarian reserve testing is the monthly fluctuation and varying length of cycles especially in the setting of diminished ovarian reserve (DOR) or POI (87).

AMH (Anti-Mullerian Hormone)

AMH historically is known for its role in male in-utero sexual development, causing Mullerian duct regression. In the ovaries, AMH is produced by the granulosa cells in growing ovarian follicles, from the primary stage to the small antral stage. There is then decreased expression due to the FSH-dependent selection process, with some continued expression in the cumulus cells of pre-ovulatory follicles. AMH is not present in atretic follicles or corpora lutea (88). Clinically, AMH is used to help predict response to ovarian response to COH (89); however, it has not shown to be as useful in predicting pregnancy or live birth (90–93).

Measuring serum AMH levels prior to cancer treatment can serve as a baseline comparison of ovarian reserve to AMH after treatment completion (94, 95). One study found that women with higher AMH levels pre chemotherapy maintained higher levels after treatment, while those with lower initial levels experienced a more gradual recovery of AMH levels (96). Moreover, for breast cancer patients, combining pre-treatment AMH levels with age significantly enhances the accuracy of predicting cancer therapy-induced amenorrhea, offering valuable insights into ovarian function post treatment (88).

AMH is more frequently being obtained prior to cancer treatment and in survivorship to study the effects of ovarian reserve. One study revealed that the older a patient is at the time of their cancer diagnosis, the more significant the expected reduction in AMH levels post-treatment (97). A Dutch longitudinal study monitored AMH levels in 192 childhood cancer survivors for an average of 3.2 years post treatment (98). At their first assessment, these survivors' AMH levels were 0.59 μg/L below the median for their age, and at a follow-up visit 3.2 years later, the levels were 0.22 μg/L below the median for their age. However, those who regained ovarian function and had an AMH over 1 μg/L did not show a faster decline in AMH compared to their healthy counterparts. Nearly 40% of those with initial AMH levels below 1 μg/L experienced an increase in AMH to above 1 μg/L within 3.2 years. These results offer some optimism for child and AYA survivors, though further research is needed to understand the long-term implications as these individuals enter their 30s and 40s (98). A systematic review done by Anderson et al. analyzed AMH levels before, during, and after cancer treatment and took into consideration a patient's age and treatment regimen. Figure 7.2 represents a schematic of three general paths of AMH decline and recovery and risk of POI that may occur as a result of gonadotoxic cancer treatment (95, 99).

AFC (Antral Follicle Count)

AFC also assesses ovarian reserve by measuring the number of follicles 2–10 mm in diameter on ultrasound (usually transvaginal). Measurements are the mean diameter in two dimensions. It is

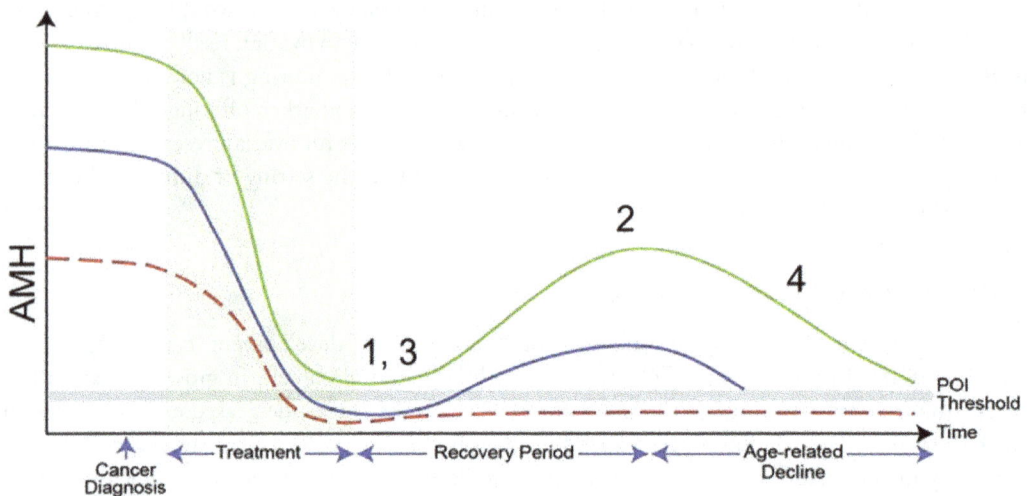

Figure 7.2   Schematic of changes in AMH as a biomarker of ovarian reserve and POI before, during, and after cancer treatment.

Reproduced from Anderson et al. (2022) (95) with permission, modified from Jayasinghe et al (2018) (99)

often performed on menstrual cycle days two through four and has low intercycle variability and high reliability in experienced centers (100). Limitations of this method are based on quality of the ultrasound images and skill of the ultrasound technician (101). Similar to AMH, AFC has been shown to be sensitive and specific to predict ovarian response to COH (89, 102), but is limited in pregnancy rates and live birth rates (100).

Assessing Fertility after Cancer Treatment

Navigating the complexities of fertility after cancer treatment presents both challenges and hopeful opportunities for survivors. Because cancer therapies can significantly impact reproductive health, understanding and addressing post-treatment fertility is crucial. This includes evaluating how different types of cancer and their treatments, such as chemotherapy, radiation, or surgery, influence fertility potential. Advances in reproductive medicine offer various options for cancer survivors, ranging from the use of cryopreserved embryos to assisted reproductive technologies. Additionally, there is growing importance in counseling and support services to help survivors understand their fertility options and make informed decisions. There are currently minimal guidelines regarding post-treatment assessment of fertility for AYA cancer survivors. The majority of fertility assessment recommendations are regarding care pre treatment or with recurrence.

Pubertal Status

Though the 2020 Oncofertility Pediatric Interest Network's female risk stratification system was created to help counsel patients on fertility preservation options prior to chemotherapy and/ or radiation (103), it can also to help counsel and guide monitoring in survivorship by evaluating the cancer treatment received. The risk stratification was based on expert opinion and literature review to assess the patient's risk for premature ovarian insufficiency from gonadotoxicity level of the cancer treatment. It incorporates pubertal status, cyclophosphamide equivalent dose (CED), and radiation dose and location. Risk for gonadotoxicity is separated into three risk groups: minimally increased risk, significantly increased risk, and high level of increased risk. This stratification system was recently validated by a mega-analysis using AMH levels in cancer survivors (104).

Postpubertal

After cancer treatment is complete, it is not uncommon for patients to have amenorrhea for a few months. It can sometimes take one to two years for menses to return (107). However, it is important to note that survivors with regular menstrual cycles post treatment may still be at risk of POI and infertility. While menstrual regularity is an important sign, it should not be solely relied on to assess ovarian reserve in this population. A study of 100 pediatric cancer survivors diagnosed before age 15 and off treatment for a year revealed that 70% had regular periods, but the overall cohort exhibited lower early follicular phase estradiol and antral follicle count compared to their peers. Over a ten-year follow-up, these patients generally had preserved ovarian function into their mid-thirties (108). Women who had undergone pelvic radiation or treatment with alkylating agents experienced greater impairment of ovarian reserve and faced more challenges with conception (109).

There currently are no recommendations regarding survivorship fertility surveillance in adult women, AMH level monitoring, or when to refer for post-treatment fertility preservation. The authors of this chapter recommend monitoring FSH, LH, estradiol, and AMH annually starting one year after cancer treatment is complete. If a patient is experiencing irregular menses, secondary amenorrhea, sexual function changes, or clinical signs of estrogen deficiency such as hot flashes, or if there is exposure to alkylating agents or pelvic radiation, the patient should be referred to an OB/GYN or reproductive endocrinologist for further evaluation. Cancer survivors can be counseled on post-treatment fertility preservation options, risk of POI, and hormone replacement if indicated.

Ovarian Function Status

Diminished Ovarian Reserve (DOR)

Diminished ovarian reserve (DOR) is a significant concern in reproductive medicine, referring to a condition in which the ovaries have fewer oocytes available for fertilization than would be expected for a woman's age. It is a critical factor affecting fertility, since it not only impacts the chances of conception but also influences the response to fertility treatments. While normal aging is the most common inciting factor, DOR can also result from genetic causes, chemotherapy, surgeries involving the ovaries, and lifestyle factors such as smoking (110).

There is no current consensus on a definition for DOR; however, in clinical practice a modified Bologna Criteria for poor ovarian response to hyperstimulation has been utilized. This includes women with normal menstrual cycles exhibiting low AMH levels (less than 0.5–1.1 ng/mL), reduced antral follicle count (less than 5–7), and/or high, but non-menopausal FSH levels (10–25 mIU/mL) (111, 112). In pediatric research, an AMH level below the fifth percentile for age has been used for abnormally low ovarian reserve, though the implication for future fertility is not well understood, and pregnancy outcomes require further research (113).

Premature Ovarian Insufficiency (POI)

While DOR refers to a decrease in the quantity and quality of remaining oocytes, premature ovarian insufficiency (POI) is a condition in which the ovaries cease to function normally before the age of 40. Primary ovarian insufficiency and premature ovarian insufficiency are often used interchangeably, but the authors' preferred term is premature ovarian insufficiency in agreement with the European Society for Human Reproduction and Embryology (ESHRE) guidelines (114). POI in individuals who have undergone cancer treatment can result from the adverse effects of chemotherapy and radiation on ovarian follicles (115, 116). This condition presents as amenorrhea or oligomenorrhea, or menopausal symptoms, due to decreased ovarian function before the age 40 (117, 118). While there is no consensus in diagnosis for POI, the American College of Obstetricians and Gynecologists (ACOG) recommends workup if experiencing irregular menses for three months, evaluation of FSH and estradiol one month apart, and evaluation for other hormonal causes (e.g., hypothyroidism, hyperprolactinemia) that could lead to amenorrhea (119). Clinically, patients may also present with vasomotor symptoms, night sweats, vaginal dryness, or irritability (118, 120). If the initial test shows FSH levels in the menopausal range (generally above 25–40 mIU/mL), a repeat FSH test should be conducted after one month. A consistent finding of elevated FSH on this second test is consistent with a POI diagnosis. Estradiol levels below 50 pg/mL are indicative of low estrogen levels, or hypoestrogenism (121, 122). While AMH has been established as a marker of ovarian reserve and has been suggested to be of importance in the diagnosis of POI, it is often undetectable; thus, further investigation is required to make a diagnosis of POI (95).

After the diagnosis of POI, further workup should be done to determine a potential cause (e.g., anti-thyroid and anti-adrenal antibodies for autoimmune oophoritis, Fragile X testing for the premutation, and karyotype for Turner Syndrome). Additionally, after the diagnosis, spontaneous conception and pregnancy have been noted, and rates range from 2% to as high as 14% likely due to intermittent ovarian functioning (119, 123). Of note, the hypoestrogenic state due to POI can lead to reduced bone density and osteoporosis, cardiovascular disease, genitourinary symptoms of menopause, and changes in cognition (124), and these are addressed in detail in other chapters.

Acute POI, Persistent POI, Late POI

Acute POI, also termed acute ovarian failure (AOF), is defined by the St. Jude's Childhood Cancer Survivor Study as primary amenorrhea after cancer treatment (if diagnosed prior to menarche) or permanent loss of ovarian function resulting in secondary amenorrhea within five years after cancer treatment (if diagnosed after menarche) (125, 126). An online calculator tool has been created to estimate the risk of AOF based on age and treatment. Of note, the calculator does not predict long-term POI (127). Similar to POI, there is a drop in estrogen levels, rise in FSH levels, and low/undetectable AMH levels causing amenorrhea or absence of puberty. Acute POI in childhood cancer survivors has been reported between 6.3% and 12% (82, 128). The CCSS identified an elevated risk if radiation to the ovaries was greater than 1000 cGy and if alkylating chemotherapy (e.g., procarbazine and cyclophosphamide) was used (83). Studies have shown that it may take up to two or three years for AMH levels to recover to a new baseline after cancer treatment (129). If acute POI does not have recovery of ovarian function, patients may then have persistent POI. However, those who do have ovarian function recovery may still be at risk for diminished ovarian reserve (DOR) and late POI later in life (Figure 7.1).

Radiotherapy: Disruption of the Hypothalamic-Pituitary-Ovary (HPO) Axis, Presentation, and Management

Depending on the location of the radiation there may be different sequelae. Cranial spinal irradiation, often seen in patients with neuroblastoma, can cause infertility by disrupting the HPO axis leading to a deficiency in gonadotropins (130–133). Patients may present with primary or secondary amenorrhea, and hormone evaluations may show low FSH, low LH, and low estradiol with normal/detectable AMH. This type of infertility is different because ovarian reserve and function have not been compromised by gonadotoxic therapy. Instead, the communication to stimulate the ovaries has been disrupted. Fertility can potentially be restored with the use of exogenous gonadotropins to induce ovulation similarly to patients with hypothalamic hypogonadism due to other causes (134, 135).

Radiotherapy: Effects on the Uterus, Presentation, and Management

Uterine radiation can effect uterine function and fertility in terms of implantation (15). This may result in several clinical presentations. Patients may present with primary or secondary amenorrhea and normal gonadotropin and estradiol levels. Amenorrhea is due to the endometrium not proliferating appropriately (136, 137). Some patients may not experience a withdrawal bleed even after a Provera challenge (i.e., 10 mg of medroxyprogesterone acetate for ten days). A history of pelvic or whole-body irradiation and imaging with a reduced uterine size or a thin endometrial lining can help with the diagnosis of uterine factor infertility due to radiation. Underdeveloped uteri may be present in patients who received pelvic radiation prior to puberty (138). Patients with this diagnosis can benefit from a fertility referral, counseling about surrogacy, and may be appropriate candidates to consider uterine transplantation. Uterine transplantation is still considered experimental in the United States with the first live birth in 2014 (139, 140).

Fertility Preservation after Cancer Treatment

Ideally discussions about cancer treatment and reproductive effects and fertility preservation options should be offered to patients prior to treatment initiation. However, patients who do not have time, were not counseled, had limited access, or had limited funds for fertility preservation prior to cancer treatment should be counseled and given information during survivorship, especially if there is concern for decreased ovarian function. Both the ASRM and the ASCO have recommendations for fertility-specific counseling post cancer treatment (98). The main option is oocyte/embryo cryopreservation, which requires spontaneous menarche (if cancer treatment was prepubertal) or return of menstrual cycles (if cancer treatment was postmenarchal). However, if a patient has POI and the FSH level is >20 mIU/mL, it is unlikely ovarian hyperstimulation will be successful. One study of adolescents and young adults who underwent oocyte cryopreservation performed a sub-analysis comparing those with prior chemotherapy exposure to those without and respectively found a median AMH of 0.6 vs. 2.32 ng/mL and median number of 4 vs. 13 cryopreserved mature oocytes (43). Thus, those post treatment or with cancer relapse may have worse outcomes than if oocyte cryopreservation was done prior to chemotherapy or radiation. Given that there is more than a 30% likelihood of fertility loss due to the treatment, fertility is optimized if preservation options occur prior to treatment initiation (141).

Another study by Su et al. delved into the long-term trajectory of AMH following cancer treatment, spanning over two decades. It revealed that AMH typically takes about 1–3 years to recover to a new baseline post treatment, followed by a stabilization phase lasting around 15 years before eventually declining. Notably, patients in their late 20s had decreased recovery compared to patients younger than 25, presumed to be a result of lower ovarian reserve. Furthermore, those who underwent treatments with low or moderate gonadotoxicity showed a significant recuperation in AMH levels compared to those subjected to high toxicity treatments. These findings suggest the importance of monitoring ovarian reserve after the completion of treatment, because the fertility window, although potentially shorter, may extend beyond common expectations. Therefore, patients may still be viable candidates for post-chemotherapy fertility preservation, emphasizing the need for tailored reproductive guidance and planning in cancer survivors (129). Patients should have yearly evaluations that detail their menstrual history, sexual function (vaginal dryness, libido), any menopausal symptoms, and medication use, preferably by an OB/GYN. Though there are no recommendations, it is reasonable to obtain AMH, FSH, LH, and estradiol levels every 1–2 years and refer patients to an REI for a more comprehensive ovarian reserve evaluation, especially for patients with abnormal menstrual patterns or menopausal symptoms (104). Figure 7.3 displays a proposed flow diagram for fertility assessment after gonadotoxic treatment.

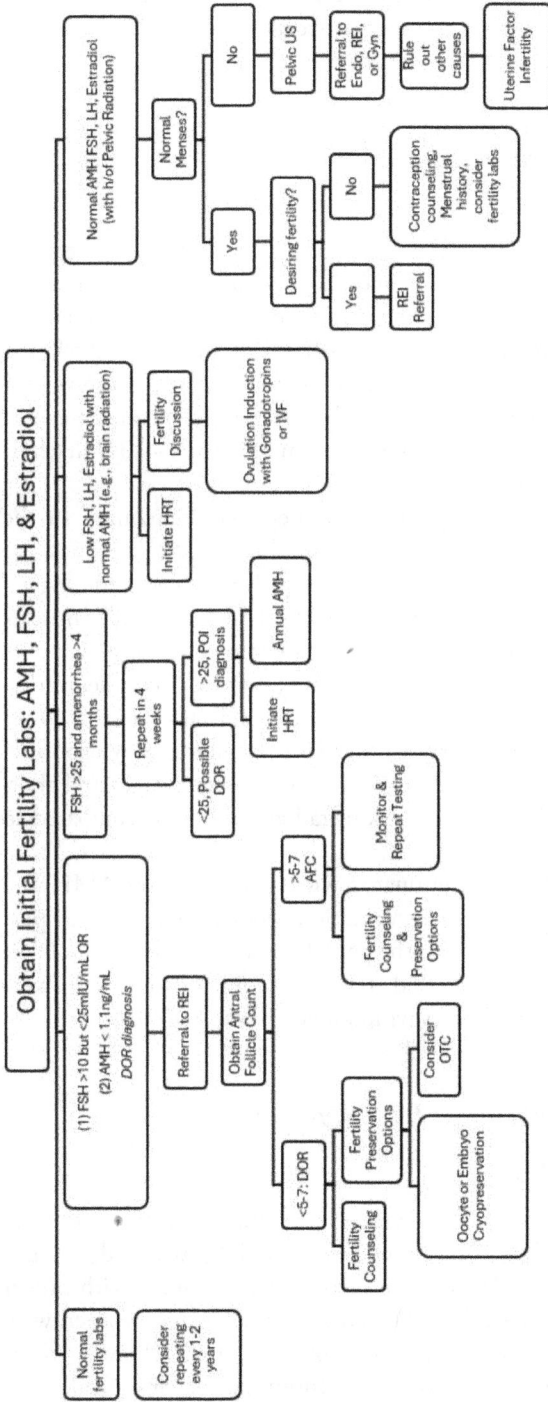

Figure 7.3   Proposed flow diagram for fertility assessment after gonadotoxic treatment. For patients who are less than 40 years old.

Acronyms: REI: Reproductive Endocrinology and Infertility, DOR: Diminished Ovarian Reserve, AMH: Anti-Mullerian Hormone, FSH: Follicle Stimulating Hormone, LH: Luteinizing hormone, AFC: Antral Follicle Count, POI: Premature ovarian insufficiency, HRT: Hormone Replacement Therapy, Gyn: Gynecology, Endo: Endocrinology, US: Ultrasound

Source: With permission, figure modified from Jayasinghe YL, Wallace WHB, Anderson RA. Ovarian function, fertility and reproductive lifespan in cancer patients. Expert Rev Endocrinol Metable 2018;13(3):125–36; Anderson RA, Cameron D, Clatot F, Demeestere I, Lambertini M, Nelson SM, Peccatori F. Anti-Müllerian hormone as a marker of ovarian reserve and premature ovarian insufficiency in children and women with cancer: a systematic review. Hum Reprod Update. 2022;28(3):417–34.

Pregnancy in Cancer Survivors

The rates of successful pregnancies differ based on whether conception is spontaneous or achieved through IVF. Moreover, the type of cancer, along with the specific treatment regimens the patient underwent, can also play a critical role in influencing pregnancy rates.

Pregnancy Rates without Fertility Preservation Interventions

A Scottish Cancer Registry of 23,201 females diagnosed with cancer before the age of 40, between 1981 and 2012, were followed until 2014 for pregnancy outcomes. Compared to the general female population, these cancer survivors had notably lower pregnancy rates of 6,627 actual pregnancies versus an expected 10,736, resulting in a Standardized Incidence Ratio (SIR) of 0.62 (95% CI: 0.60, 0.63). This suggests that cancer survivors were about 38% less likely to become pregnant post diagnosis. A significantly reduced SIR was observed across almost all types of cancer, except for liver cancer, which was relatively rare. The SIR varied, ranging from 0.34 (0.31–0.37) in cervical cancer cases to 0.87 (0.84–0.90) in skin cancer cases (142).

Different treatment regimens also contribute to spontaneous pregnancy outcomes. In the Childhood Cancer Survivor Study, for women who underwent chemotherapy only (n = 154), the RR for various pregnancy outcomes were as follows: live births had an RR of 0.52, indicating a lower likelihood compared to controls; stillbirths were relatively rare with an RR of 1.00; miscarriages had a slightly increased risk with an RR of 1.07; and the rate of abortions was notably higher with an RR of 2.47. On the other hand, in the case of radiation therapy only to either the ovaries, uterus, or hypothalamus/pituitary, the number of pregnancies reported was considerably lower (n = 5). The outcomes included an RR of 0.52 for live births, similar to chemotherapy exposure. However, there were no stillbirths reported in this group, and the RR for miscarriages and abortions were 1.73 and 1.81 respectively, suggesting a higher risk of radiation therapy compared to chemotherapy alone (126).

In a mega-analysis of cancer survivors who were evaluated with post-treatment AMH levels, 26.9% (59/219) of patients asked about pregnancy information reported a pregnancy post treatment. Interestingly, pregnancy did not correspond to the gonadotoxicity risk level (p = 0.70) of their cancer treatment (104). In women who conceived, the most common diagnoses were Hodgkin's lymphoma (55.9%; 33/59) and non-Hodgkin's lymphoma (18.6%; 11/59).

Pregnancy Rates with Fertility Preservation Interventions

Oocytes/Embryos

Meernik et al. conducted a meta-analysis and systematic review comparing assisted reproductive technology (ART) outcomes between women with and without cancer. They analyzed 42 studies across various countries from 1995 to 2020. There was a median of 58 women with cancer and 114 women without cancer per study. The study indicated that, on average, women with cancer were less likely to return for embryo transfer and had lower odds of achieving clinical pregnancy and live birth after ART compared to women without cancer. Specifically, the odds ratio (OR) for clinical pregnancy was 0.51 (95% CI: 0.35, 0.73) and for live birth was

0.56 (95% CI: 0.38, 0.83), suggesting a reduced likelihood of these outcomes in women with a cancer history (143).

Ovarian Tissue Transplantation

An ovarian tissue transplantation (OTT) occurs when the patient is ready to attempt pregnancy. While OTC is a relatively new clinical option, it has resulted in over 200 live births as of 2017 (45, 144–146). The pregnancy rate has been described as 18–50%, live birth rate of 23–41%, 33–55% of the live births were conceived spontaneously after tissue transplant, and the remaining required assisted reproductive techniques or data was not available (145, 147, 148). Of note, only two successful live births have occurred from prepubertal/peripubertal tissue (149, 150), both of whom were not cancer patients. It is possibly because many of these young girls have not yet reached an age to start family building or have not returned to use their tissue.

Comparison of Techniques

Within patients who had fertility preservation prior to cancer treatment, there are varying live birth rates by fertility preservation method. A 2022 meta-analysis evaluated live birth rates for patients after cancer treatment or bone marrow transplant and compared live birth rates after: (1) embryo transfer after embryo cryopreservation (41%) (n = 175), (2) embryo transfer after oocyte cryopreservation and IVF (32%) (n = 177), (3) spontaneous pregnancies after OTC and OTT (33%) (n = 342), (4) IVF after OTC and OTT (21%) (n = 266). A limitation of this study was the diversity of patient population and study type; however, it allows for a comparison of live birth rates across the four different main fertility preservation options (151).

Long-Term Monitoring by Oncologist, Gynecologist, or REI

The primary method of fertility preservation for cancer survivors largely focuses on oocyte or embryo cryopreservation before the onset of POI. This is followed by long-term monitoring, which includes tracking the regularity of menstrual cycles, fertility status, and raising awareness about family building options. Often, those who continue to experience normal menstrual cycles after treatment tend to discontinue follow-up, operating under the assumption that their fertility has remained unaffected by their cancer or its treatment.

Given the increased rates of POI and earlier onset of DOR, we advocate for regular fertility monitoring in those who are younger than 40 or those who are still interested in future fertility. We recommend routine monitoring of AMH, FSH, LH, and estradiol every one to two years after treatment completion. If abnormal, recommend prompt referral to REI if there is concern for diminished ovarian reserve and further workup in one month if suggestive of POI. While there is evidence that AMH can be used as a marker for ovarian function in this population, there is currently no recommended standard of care for screening in this population (95) or the meaning of its value, especially in prepubertal girls. Further research should focus on the efficacy of long-term monitoring to diagnose POI, DOR, and impact on long-term health. See Figure 7.3 for further breakdown of a possible monitoring algorithm.

CASE PRESENTATIONS

Case scenario 1: *A 19-year-old female, diagnosed with Ewing sarcoma in her right leg at age 5 and treated with chemotherapy including vincristine, doxorubicin, and cyclophosphamide, presents for a well-woman visit with her primary care physician. She received a cyclophosphamide equivalent dose (CED) of 8,400 mg/m². She underwent spontaneous puberty at 11 years old and menarche at 13 years old and has had regular menstrual cycles. She did not undergo any fertility preservation procedures prior to treatment.*

    Discussion: Given this patient's history of chemoradiation treatment, she is at an increased risk of premature ovarian insufficiency (POI). Consider the following in today's visit:

- Obtain detailed menstrual cycle and sexual history.
- Consider monitoring of anti-Mullerian hormone (AMH) and follicle-stimulating hormone (FSH) to assess ovarian reserve. But counsel patent on the limitations of the utility of the AMH level and that it cannot predict future fertility, pregnancy loss, or age of menopause. More data and research are needed in this patient population (100, 152). See Figure 7.3.
- Of note, cyclophosphamide equivalent dose (CED) is a method used to standardize the doses of various chemotherapy drugs to a common measure for comparison purposes. The calculation of CED is based on the concept that different chemotherapeutic agents have different potencies and mechanisms of action, and thus their doses cannot be directly compared. The CED is calculated using specific conversion factors for each drug, which are derived from their relative toxicities compared to cyclophosphamide. The calculator can be found at https://www.oncofertilityrisk.com/CED.html (153). Doses of chemotherapy drugs should be noted in patient's oncology records.
- Based on the 2020 Oncofertility Network Pediatric Initiative Network Risk Stratification table (154), she was prepubertal and CED >8,000 mg/m² at the time of cancer treatment, putting her in the "increased risk" level for gonadotoxicity.
- Assess family planning and fertility goals.

  - Counsel patient on egg freezing if desire to have children in the future is expressed and has hormone levels concerning for diminished ovarian reserve.
  - Counsel about contraception option if pregnancy is not desired.

Case scenario 2: *A 30-year-old female with a history of lymphoma treated with a hematopoietic stem cell transplant presents to the clinic after being amenorrheic for five months and experiencing recurrent hot flashes. She reports that her menstrual cycles were previously regular, occurring every 28 days, with a duration of 3–5 days. She has never been pregnant but is interested in conceiving.*

    Discussion: This patient needs to be evaluated for primary ovarian insufficiency. Consider the following in today's visit:

- Rule out pregnancy with a serum hCG measurement.
- Obtain FSH, LH, estradiol, AMH, TSH, Free T4, and prolactin levels.

- If the initial test shows FSH levels in the menopausal range (generally above 25–40 mIU/mL), a repeat FSH test should be conducted after one month. A consistent finding of elevated FSH on this second test is consistent with a POI diagnosis.
- Counsel patient on egg donation if pregnancy is strongly desired and refer to a reproductive endocrinology and infertility specialist. Discuss with the patient that there is a low but possible ~5% chance of conceiving naturally.
- If patient does not wish to become pregnant, she should be counseled on contraceptive options.
- Counsel patient on needing hormone replacement therapy (HRT) until ~50 years old for bone, cardiovascular, and cognitive health. Options can include 0.1 mg transdermal 17 β estradiol or 2 mg of oral 17 β estradiol PLUS oral progestin (cyclical or continuous oral Prometrium or medroxyprogesterone acetate) (155) or levonorgestrel intrauterine device. An alternative is a continuous combined oral contraceptive pill with 30 mcg or more of ethinyl estradiol for bone health. It is important that regardless of HRT the patient is on a continuous dose of estrogen.

Conclusion

Cancer treatments including chemotherapy and radiation put survivors at increased risk for DOR and POI. The main goal is to give patients information and autonomy to make choices about if or how they want to build their family in the future. Thus, risk of gonadotoxicity and fertility preservation options should be offered before and after cancer treatment. Additionally, menstrual cycle and serum ovarian reserve monitoring should be universally available to all cancer survivors, irrespective of the type of cancer or the specifics of their treatment plan. Survivors can then be referred to a specialist for additional counseling and evaluation if needed. Counseling should be tailored to each individual patient encompassing nuances such as patient's age, duration since completing treatment, the gonadotoxic effects of the therapy received, indicators of ovarian reserve, and their fertility desires.

References

1. Group USCSW. U.S. Cancer Statistics Data Visualizations Tool: U.S. Department of Health and Human Services, Centers for Disease Control and Prevention and National Cancer Institute [updated June 2024]. Available from: https://www.cdc.gov/cancer/dataviz.
2. Phillips SM et al. Survivors of childhood cancer in the United States: Prevalence and burden of morbidity. Cancer Epidemiol Biomarkers Prev. 2015;24(4):653–63.
3. Wu Y et al. Global, regional, and national childhood cancer burden, 1990–2019: An analysis based on the Global Burden of Disease Study 2019. J Adv Res. 2022;40:233–47.
4. Koh B et al. Patterns in cancer incidence among people younger than 50 years in the US, 2010 to 2019. JAMA Netw Open. 2023;6(8):e2328171.
5. Zhang S et al. Chemotherapy impairs ovarian function through excessive ROS-induced ferroptosis. Cell Death Dis. 2023;14(5):340.
6. Bedoschi G et al. Chemotherapy-induced damage to ovary: Mechanisms and clinical impact. Future Oncol. 2016;12(20):2333–44.
7. Meirow D et al. Cortical fibrosis and blood-vessels damage in human ovaries exposed to chemotherapy: Potential mechanisms of ovarian injury. Hum Reprod. 2007;22(6):1626–33.

8. Hao X et al. Ovarian follicle depletion induced by chemotherapy and the investigational stages of potential fertility-protective treatments—A review. Int J Molec Sci. 2019;20(19):4720.

9. Waimey KE et al. Understanding fertility in young female cancer patients. J Women's Health. 2015;24(10):812–18.

10. Fertility Preservation Program in Pittsburgh. Cyclophosphamide Equivalent Dose (CED) Calculator. Available from: https://fertilitypreservationpittsburgh.org/fertility-resources/fertility-risk-calculator/.

11. Grigsby PW et al. Late injury of cancer therapy on the female reproductive tract. Int J Radiat Oncol Biol Phys. 1995;31(5):1281–99.

12. Biedka M et al. Fertility impairment in radiotherapy. Contemp Oncol. 2016;20(3):199–204.

13. Green DM et al. Pregnancy outcome after treatment for Wilms tumor: A report from the national Wilms tumor long-term follow-up study. J Clin Oncol. 2010;28(17):2824–30.

14. Norwitz ER et al. Placenta percreta and uterine rupture associated with prior whole body radiation therapy. Obstet Gynecol. 2001;98(5 Pt 2):929–31.

15. Teh WT et al. The impact of uterine radiation on subsequent fertility and pregnancy outcomes. Biomed Res Int. 2014;2014:1–8.

16. Wo JY, Viswanathan AN. Impact of radiotherapy on fertility, pregnancy, and neonatal outcomes in female cancer patients. Int J Radiat Oncol Biol Phys. 2009;73(5):1304–12.

17. Bath LE et al. Ovarian and uterine characteristics after total body irradiation in childhood and adolescence: Response to sex steroid replacement. Br J Obstet Gynaecol. 1999;106(12):1265–72.

18. Larsen EC et al. Radiotherapy at a young age reduces uterine volume of childhood cancer survivors. Acta Obstet Gynecol Scand. 2004;83(1):96–102.

19. Holm K et al. Ultrasound B-mode changes in the uterus and ovaries and Doppler changes in the uterus after total body irradiation and allogeneic bone marrow transplantation in childhood. Bone Marrow Transplant. 1999;23(3):259–63.

20. Practice Committee of the American Society for Reproductive Medicine. Fertility preservation in patients undergoing gonadotoxic therapy or gonadectomy: A committee opinion. Fertil Steril. 2019;112(6):1022–33.

21. Loren AW et al. Fertility preservation for patients with cancer: American Society of Clinical Oncology clinical practice guideline update. J Clin Oncol. 2013;31(19):2500–10.

22. Anderson RA et al. ESHRE guideline: Female fertility preservation. Hum Reprod Open. 2020;2020(4):hoaa052.

23. Irene Su H et al. Oncofertility. Cancer J. 2018;24(6):328–35.

24. Donnez J, Dolmans MM. Fertility preservation in women. N Engl J Med. 2017;377(17):1657–65.

25. Petropanagos A et al. Social egg freezing: Risk, benefits and other considerations. Can Med Assoc J. 2015;187(9):666–9.

26. Himpe J et al. The impact of systemic oncological treatments on the fertility of adolescents and young adults-a systematic review. Life (Basel). 2023;13(5).

27. Fabiani C et al. Oocyte quality assessment in breast cancer: Implications for fertility preservation. Cancers (Basel). 2022;14(22).

28. Di Meglio A et al. Impact of Systemic Anticancer Therapy on Fertility. Springer International Publishing; 2020: 67–80.

29. Humaidan P et al. Preventing ovarian hyperstimulation syndrome: Guidance for the clinician. Fertil Steril. 2010;94(2):389–400.

30. Kim JH et al. Outcomes of fertility preservation for female cancer patients in a single tertiary center. Yonsei Med J. 2023;64(8):497.

31. Rienzi L et al. Oocyte, embryo and blastocyst cryopreservation in ART: Systematic review and meta-analysis comparing slow-freezing versus vitrification to produce evidence for the development of global guidance. Hum Reprod Update. 2017;23(2):139–55.

32. Sönmezer M et al. Random start ovarian stimulation before gonadotoxic therapies in women with cancer: A systematic review and meta-analysis. Reprod Biomed Online. 2023;47(6):103337.

33. Del-Pozo-Lérida S et al. Preservation of fertility in patients with cancer (review). Oncol Rep. 2019;41(5):2607–14.

34. A review of best practices of rapid-cooling vitrification for oocytes and embryos: A committee opinion. Fertil Steril. 2021;115(2):305–10.
35. Rivas Leonel EC et al. Cryopreservation of human ovarian tissue: A review. Transfus Med Hemotherapy. 2019;46(3):173–81.
36. Iussig B et al. A brief history of oocyte cryopreservation: Arguments and facts. Acta Obstet Gynecol Scand. 2019;98(5):550–8.
37. Konc J et al. Cryopreservation of embryos and oocytes in human assisted reproduction. Biomed Res Int. 2014;2014:1–9.
38. Zenzes MT et al. Effects of chilling to 0 degrees C on the morphology of meiotic spindles in human metaphase II oocytes. Fertil Steril. 2001;75(4):769–77.
39. Pickering SJ et al. Transient cooling to room temperature can cause irreversible disruption of the meiotic spindle in the human oocyte. Fertil Steril. 1990;54(1):102–8.
40. Barritt J et al. Report of four donor-recipient oocyte cryopreservation cycles resulting in high pregnancy and implantation rates. Fertil Steril. 2007;87(1):189.e13–17.
41. Cobo A, Diaz C. Clinical application of oocyte vitrification: A systematic review and meta-analysis of randomized controlled trials. Fertil Steril. 2011;96(2):277–85.
42. Ho JR et al. A comparison of live birth rates and perinatal outcomes between cryopreserved oocytes and cryopreserved embryos. J Assist Reprod Genet. 2017;34(10):1359–66.
43. Manuel SL et al. Ovarian stimulation is a safe and effective fertility preservation option in the adolescent and young adult population. J Assist Reprod Genet. 2020;37(3):699–708.
44. Demeestere I et al. Live birth after autograft of ovarian tissue cryopreserved during childhood. Hum Reprod. 2015;30(9):2107–9.
45. Dolmans MM, Donnez J. Fertility preservation in women for medical and social reasons: Oocytes vs ovarian tissue. Best Pract Res Clin Obstet Gynaecol. 2021;70:63–80.
46. Donnez J et al. Ovarian cortex transplantation: Time to move on from experimental studies to open clinical application. Fertil Steril. 2015;104(5):1097–8.
47. Practice Committees of the American Society for Reproductive Medicine, the Society of Reproductive Biologists and Technologists, and the Society for Assisted Reproductive Technology. In vitro maturation: A committee opinion. Fertil Steril. 2021;115(2):298–304.
48. Corkum KS et al. A review of reported surgical techniques in fertility preservation for prepubertal and adolescent females facing a fertility threatening diagnosis or treatment. Am J Surg. 2017;214(4):695–700.
49. Long J et al. Ovarian tissue cryopreservation of a prepubertal patient. Radiother Oncol. 2024.
50. Donnez J, Dolmans MM. Fertility preservation in women. Nat Rev Endocrinol. 2013;9(12):735–49.
51. Sugishita Y et al. Comparison of open and a novel closed vitrification system with slow freezing for human ovarian tissue cryopreservation. J Assist Reprod Genet. 2021;38(10):2723–33.
52. Son W-Y et al. Immature oocyte for fertility preservation. Front Endocrinol. 2019;10.
53. Barahmeh S et al. Ovarian transposition before pelvic irradiation: Indications and functional outcome. J Obstet Gynaecol Res. 2013;39(11):1533–7.
54. Morice P et al. Fertility results after ovarian transposition for pelvic malignancies treated by external irradiation or brachytherapy. Hum Reprod. 1998;13(3):660–3.
55. Blumenfeld Z. How to preserve fertility in young women exposed to chemotherapy? The role of GnRH agonist cotreatment in addition to cryopreservation of embrya, oocytes, or ovaries. Oncologist. 2007;12:1044–54.
56. Blumenfeld Z. GnRH-agonists in fertility preservation. Curr Opin Endocrinol Diabetes Obes. 2008;15(6):523–8.
57. Yu B, Davidson NE. Gonadotropin-Releasing Hormone (GnRH) agonists for fertility preservation: Is POEMS the final verse? JNCI. 2019;111(2):107–8.
58. Elgindy EA et al. Gonadotrophin suppression to prevent chemotherapy-induced ovarian damage: A randomized controlled trial. Obstet Gynecol. 2013;121(1):78–86.
59. Demeestere I et al. No evidence for the benefit of gonadotropin-releasing hormone agonist in preserving ovarian function and fertility in lymphoma survivors treated with chemotherapy: Final long-term report of a prospective randomized trial. J Clin Oncol. 2016;34(22):2568–74.

60. Blumenfeld Z. Fertility preservation using GnRH agonists: Rationale, possible mechanisms, and explanation of controversy. Clin Med Insights: Reprod Health. 2019;13:117955811987016.
61. Valsamakis G et al. GnRH analogues as a co-treatment to therapy in women of reproductive age with cancer and fertility preservation. Int J Molec Sci. 2022;23(4):2287.
62. Moawad NS et al. Laparoscopic ovarian transposition before pelvic cancer treatment: Ovarian function and fertility preservation. J Minim Invasive Gynecol. 2017;24(1):28–35.
63. Bisharah M, Tulandi T. Laparoscopic preservation of ovarian function: An underused procedure. Am J Obstet Gynecol. 2003;188(2):367–70.
64. Fisch B, Abir R. Female fertility preservation: Past, present and future. Reproduction. 2018;156(1):F11–27.
65. Arian SE et al. Ovarian transposition: A surgical option for fertility preservation. Fertil Steril. 2017;107(4):e15.
66. Ribeiro R et al. Uterine transposition: Technique and a case report. Fertil Steril. 2017;108(2):320–4.e1.
67. Ribeiro R et al. Uterine transposition technique: Update and review. Minerva Ginecol. 2019;71(1):62–71.
68. Pavone M et al. Uterine transposition versus uterine ventrofixation before radiotherapy as a fertility sparing option in young women with pelvic malignancies: Systematic review of the literature and dose simulation. Eur J Surg Oncol. 2024;50(1):107270.
69. Ribeiro R et al. Uterine transposition for fertility and ovarian function preservation after radiotherapy. Int J Gynecol Cancer. 2023;33(12):1837–42.
70. Batman SH, Schmeler KM. Fertility-sparing and less radical surgery for cervical cancer. Current Oncology Reports. 2022.
71. Zhao XL et al. Fertility-preserving treatment in patients with early-stage endometrial cancer: A protocol for systematic review and meta-analysis. Medicine (Baltimore). 2021;100(48):e27961.
72. Mutlu L et al. Endometrial cancer in reproductive age: Fertility-sparing approach and reproductive outcomes. Cancers (Basel). 2022;14(21).
73. Perrin LC et al. Fertility and ovarian function after conservative surgery for germ cell tumors of the ovary. Aust N Z J Obstet Gynaecol. 1999;39(2):243–5.
74. Lim-Tan SK et al. Ovarian cystectomy for serous borderline tumors: A follow-up study of 35 cases. Obstet Gynecol. 1988;72(5):775–81.
75. Vollenhoven B, Hunt S. Ovarian ageing and the impact on female fertility. F1000Res. 2018;7:1835.
76. American College of Obstetricians and Gynecologists Committee on Gynecologic Practice and Practice Committee. Female age-related fertility decline. Committee opinion 589. Fertil Steril. 2014;101(3):633–4.
77. Hansen KR et al. A new model of reproductive aging: The decline in ovarian non-growing follicle number from birth to menopause. Hum Reprod. 2008;23(3):699–708.
78. Wasielak-Politowska M, Kordowitzki P. Chromosome segregation in the oocyte: What goes wrong during aging. Int J Mol Sci. 2022;23(5).
79. Robison LL et al. Study design and cohort characteristics of the Childhood Cancer Survivor Study: A multi-institutional collaborative project. Med Pediatr Oncol. 2002;38(4):229–39.
80. Green DM et al. Fertility of female survivors of childhood cancer: A report from the Childhood Cancer Survivor Study. J Clin Oncol. 2009;27(16):2677–85.
81. Chow EJ et al. Pregnancy after chemotherapy in male and female survivors of childhood cancer treated between 1970 and 1999: A report from the Childhood Cancer Survivor Study cohort. Lancet Oncol. 2016;17(5):567–76.
82. Sklar CA et al. Premature menopause in survivors of childhood cancer: A report from the Childhood Cancer Survivor Study. JNCI. 2006;98(13):890–6.
83. Chemaitilly W et al. Acute ovarian failure in the Childhood Cancer Survivor Study. J Clin Endocrinol Metab. 2006;91(5):1723–8.
84. Roeca C et al. Recommendations for assessing ovarian health and fertility potential in survivors of childhood cancer. Maturitas. 2019;122:57–9.
85. Barnhart K, Osheroff J. Follicle stimulating hormone as a predictor of fertility. Curr Opin Obstet Gynecol. 1998;10(3):227–32.

86. Sharara FI et al. The detection of diminished ovarian reserve in infertile women. Am J Obstet Gynecol. 1998;179(3 Pt 1):804–12.
87. Perloe M et al. Strategies for ascertaining ovarian reserve among women suspected of subfertility. Int J Fertil Womens Med. 2000;45(3):215–24.
88. Sonigo C et al. Anti-Müllerian Hormone in fertility preservation: Clinical and therapeutic applications. Clin Med Insights: Reprod Health. 2019;13:117955811985475.
89. Broer SL et al. Added value of ovarian reserve testing on patient characteristics in the prediction of ovarian response and ongoing pregnancy: An individual patient data approach. Hum Reprod Update. 2013;19(1):26–36.
90. Zarek SM et al. Anti-Müllerian Hormone and pregnancy loss from the effects of aspirin in gestation and reproduction trial. Fertil Steril. 2016;105(4):946–52.e2.
91. Tal R et al. Anti-Müllerian Hormone as a predictor of live birth following assisted reproduction: An analysis of 85,062 fresh and thawed cycles from the society for assisted reproductive technology clinic outcome reporting system database for 2012–2013. Fertil Steril. 2018;109(2):258–65.
92. Miyagi M et al. Live birth outcomes from IVF treatments in younger patients with low AMH. JBRA Assist Reprod. 2021;25(3):417–21.
93. Hansen KR et al. Predictors of pregnancy and live-birth in couples with unexplained infertility after ovarian stimulation-intrauterine insemination. Fertil Steril. 2016;105(6):1575–83.e2.
94. Shrikhande L et al. AMH and its clinical implications. J Obstet Gynecol India. 2020;70(5):337–41.
95. Anderson RA et al. Anti-Müllerian Hormone as a marker of ovarian reserve and premature ovarian insufficiency in children and women with cancer: A systematic review. Hum Reprod Update. 2022;28(3):417–34.
96. Xu H et al. Clinical applications of serum Anti-Müllerian Hormone measurements in both males and females: An update. Innovation. 2021;2(1):100091.
97. Wong QHY, Anderson RA. The role of antimullerian hormone in assessing ovarian damage from chemotherapy, radiotherapy and surgery. Curr Opin Endocrinol Diabetes Obes. 2018;25(6):391–8.
98. Van Der Kooi ALF et al. Longitudinal follow-up in female childhood cancer survivors: No signs of accelerated ovarian function loss. Hum Reprod. 2017;32(1):193–200.
99. Jayasinghe YL et al. Ovarian function, fertility and reproductive lifespan in cancer patients. Expert Rev Endocrinol Metab. 2018;13(3):125–36.
100. Practice Committee of the American Society for Reproductive Medicine; Practice Committee of the American Society for Reproductive Medicine. Testing and interpreting measures of ovarian reserve: A committee opinion. Fertil Steril. 2020;114(6):1151–7.
101. Mutlu MF et al. Antral follicle count determines poor ovarian response better than Anti-Müllerian Hormone but age is the only predictor for live birth in in vitro fertilization cycles. J Assist Reprod Genet. 2013;30(5):657–65.
102. Broer SL et al. AMH and AFC as predictors of excessive response in controlled ovarian hyperstimulation: A meta-analysis. Hum Reprod Update. 2011;17(1):46–54.
103. Meacham LR et al. Standardizing risk assessment for treatment-related gonadal insufficiency and infertility in childhood adolescent and young adult cancer: The pediatric initiative network risk stratification system. J Adolesc Young Adult Oncol. 2020;9(6):662–6.
104. Yano Maher JC et al. A mega-analysis of Anti-Müllerian Hormone levels in female childhood cancer survivors based on treatment risk, time since treatment, and pubertal status. J Adolesc Young Adult Oncol. 2024.
105. Hudson MM et al. Long-term follow-up care for childhood, adolescent, and young adult cancer survivors. Pediatrics. 2021;148(3):e2021053127.
106. Metzger ML et al. Female reproductive health after childhood, adolescent, and young adult cancers: Guidelines for the assessment and management of female reproductive complications. J Clin Oncol. 2013;31(9):1239–47.
107. Jacobson MH et al. Menses resumption after cancer treatment–induced amenorrhea occurs early or not at all. Fertil Steril. 2016;105(3):765–72.e4.
108. Nielsen SN et al. A 10-year follow up of reproductive function in women treated for childhood cancer. Reprod Biomed Online. 2013;27(2):192–200.

109. Larsen EC et al. Reduced ovarian function in long-term survivors of radiation- and chemotherapy-treated childhood cancer. J Clin Endocrinol Metab. 2003;88(11):5307–14.

110. Zhu Q et al. Potential factors result in diminished ovarian reserve: A comprehensive review. J Ovarian Res. 2023;16(1).

111. Cohen J et al. Diminished ovarian reserve, premature ovarian failure, poor ovarian responder—a plea for universal definitions. J Assist Reprod Genet. 2015;32(12):1709–12.

112. Pastore LM et al. Reproductive ovarian testing and the alphabet soup of diagnoses: DOR, POI, POF, POR, and FOR. J Assist Reprod Genet. 2018;35(1):17–23.

113. Nickel RS et al. Fertility after curative therapy for sickle cell disease: A comprehensive review to guide care. J Clin Med. 2022;11(9).

114. Panay N, Anderson RA, Bennie A, Cedars M, Davies M, Ee C, Gravholt CH, Kalantaridou S, Kallen A, Kim KQ, Misrahi M, Mousa A, Nappi RE, Rocca WA, Ruan X, Teede H, Vermeulen N, Vogt E, Vincent AJ; ESHRE, ASRM, CREWHIRL, and IMS Guideline Group on POI. Evidence-based guideline: premature ovarian insufficiency. Hum Reprod Open. 2024 Dec 9;2024(4):hoae065. doi: 10.1093/hropen/hoae065. PMID: 39660328; PMCID: PMC11631070.

115. Pouillès JM et al. Influence of early age at menopause on vertebral bone mass. J Bone Miner Res. 1994;9(3):311–15.

116. Sullivan JM, Fowlkes LP. The clinical aspects of estrogen and the cardiovascular system. Obstet Gynecol. 1996;87(2_suppl):36s–43s.

117. Yang XP, Reckelhoff JF. Estrogen, hormonal replacement therapy and cardiovascular disease. Curr Opin Nephrol Hypertens. 2011;20(2):133–8.

118. Nelson LM. Primary ovarian insufficiency. N Engl J Med. 2009;360(6):606–14.

119. Committee opinion 605: Primary ovarian insufficiency in adolescents and young women. Obstet Gynecol. 2014 Jul;124(1):193–7. doi: 10.1097/01.AOG.0000451757.51964.98. PMID: 24945456.

120. Rebar RW. Premature ovarian "failure" in the adolescent. Ann N Y Acad Sci. 2008;1135:138–45.

121. Jiao X et al. Ovarian reserve markers in premature ovarian insufficiency: Within different clinical stages and different etiologies. Front Endocrinol. 2021;12.

122. Pederson J et al. Primary ovarian insufficiency in adolescents: A case series. Int J Pediatr Endocrinol. 2015;2015(1).

123. Fraison E et al. Pregnancy following diagnosis of premature ovarian insufficiency: A systematic review. Reprod Biomed Online. 2019;39(3):467–76.

124. Gebauer J et al. Long-term endocrine and metabolic consequences of cancer treatment: A systematic review. Endocr Rev. 2019;40(3):711–67.

125. Clark RA et al. Predicting acute ovarian failure in female survivors of childhood cancer: A cohort study in the Childhood Cancer Survivor Study (CCSS) and the St Jude Lifetime Cohort (SJLIFE). Lancet Oncol. 2020;21(3):436–45.

126. Green DM et al. Ovarian failure and reproductive outcomes after childhood cancer treatment: Results from the childhood cancer survivor study. J Clin Oncol. 2009;27(14):2374–81.

127. CCSS SJ. Ovarian Risk Calculator. Available from: https://ccss.stjude.org/resources/calculators/ovarian-risk-calculator.html.

128. Stillman RJ et al. Ovarian failure in long-term survivors of childhood malignancy. Am J Obstet Gynecol. 1981;139(1):62–6.

129. Su HI et al. Modeling variation in the reproductive lifespan of female adolescent and young adult cancer survivors using AMH. J Clin Endocrinol Metab. 2020;105(8):2740–51.

130. Marci R et al. Radiations and female fertility. Reprod Biol Endocrinol. 2018;16(1):112.

131. Weber GF. DNA Damaging Drugs. Springer International Publishing; 2015: 9–112.

132. Crowne E et al. Effect of cancer treatment on hypothalamic-pituitary function. Lancet Diabetes Endocrinol. 2015;3(7):568–76.

133. Fraietta R et al. Hypogonadotropic hypogonadism revisited. Clinics (Sao Paulo). 2013;68(1_suppl):81–8.

134. Zhu J, Chan YM. Fertility issues for patients with hypogonadotropic causes of delayed puberty. Endocrinol Metab Clin North Am. 2015;44(4):821–34.

135. Bacigalupo A et al. Defining the intensity of conditioning regimens: Working definitions. Biol Blood Marrow Transplant. 2009;15(12):1628–33.

136. Marci R et al. Radiations and female fertility. Reprod Biol Endocrinol. 2018;16(1).
137. Caretto M et al. Unique Issues in Oncological Patients: From Amenorrhea to Fertility Preservation. Springer International Publishing; 2024: 141–65.
138. Larsen EC et al. Radiotherapy at a young age reduces uterine volume of childhood cancer survivors. Acta Obstet Gynecol Scand. 2004;83(1):96–102.
139. American society for reproductive medicine position statement on uterus transplantation: A committee opinion. Fertil Steril. 2018;110(4):605–10.
140. Brännström M et al. Uterus transplantation: From research, through human trials and into the future. Human Reprod Update. 2023;29(5):521–44.
141. Kim SS et al. Recommendations for fertility preservation in patients with lymphoma, leukemia, and breast cancer. J Assist Reprod Genet. 2012;29(6):465–8.
142. Anderson RA et al. The impact of cancer on subsequent chance of pregnancy: A population-based analysis. Human Reprod. 2018;33(7):1281–90.
143. Meernik C et al. Outcomes after assisted reproductive technology in women with cancer: A systematic review and meta-analysis. Human Reprod. 2023;38(1):30–45.
144. Andersen ST et al. Ovarian stimulation and assisted reproductive technology outcomes in women transplanted with cryopreserved ovarian tissue: A systematic review. Fertil Steril. 2019;112(5):908–21.
145. Gellert SE et al. Transplantation of frozen-thawed ovarian tissue: An update on worldwide activity published in peer-reviewed papers and on the Danish cohort. J Assist Reprod Genet. 2018;35(4):561–70.
146. Dolmans MM et al. Fertility preservation: The challenge of freezing and transplanting ovarian tissue. Trends Mol Med. 2021;27(8):777–91.
147. Shapira M et al. Evaluation of ovarian tissue transplantation: Results from three clinical centers. Fertil Steril. 2020;114(2):388–97.
148. Diaz-Garcia C et al. Oocyte vitrification versus ovarian cortex transplantation in fertility preservation for adult women undergoing gonadotoxic treatments: A prospective cohort study. Fertil Steril. 2018;109(3):478–85.e2.
149. Ginsburg ES et al. In vitro fertilization for cancer patients and survivors. Fertil Steril. 2001;75(4):705–10.
150. Yang Z-Y, Chian R-C. Development of in vitro maturation techniques for clinical applications. Fertil Steril. 2017;108(4):577–84.
151. Fraison E et al. Live birth rate after female fertility preservation for cancer or hematopoietic stem cell transplantation: A systematic review and meta-analysis of the three main techniques; embryo, oocyte and ovarian tissue cryopreservation. Hum Reprod. 2023;38(3):489–502.
152. ACOG committee opinion no. 773 summary: The use of AntiMüllerian Hormone in women not seeking fertility care. Obstet Gynecol. 2019 Apr;133(4):840–1. doi:10.1097/AOG.0000000000003163. PMID: 30913192.
153. Green DM et al. The cyclophosphamide equivalent dose as an approach for quantifying alkylating agent exposure: A report from the Childhood Cancer Survivor Study. Pediatr Blood Cancer. 2014;61(1):53–67.
154. Meacham LR et al. Standardizing risk assessment for treatment-related gonadal insufficiency and infertility in childhood adolescent and young adult cancer: The pediatric initiative network risk stratification system. J Adolesc Young Adult Oncol. 2020;9(6):662–6.
155. Committee opinion no. 698: Hormone therapy in primary ovarian insufficiency. Obstet Gynecol. 2017;129(5):e134–41.

Chapter 8

Breast Cancer and Symptom Management

Hana R. Rosenow, Charles L. Loprinzi and Daniel S. Childs

Menopausal Symptoms in Breast Cancer Patients

Many patients with breast cancer will experience menopausal symptoms, including hot flashes, night sweats, genitourinary symptoms, emotional irritability, and sexual dysfunction (1). We recognize that this population includes gender-diverse individuals and transgender men. However, the published evidence refers to people collectively experiencing menopause as women and does not clarify how findings might apply to the specific needs of gender-diverse individuals; thus, we will refer to the patients as women for the purpose of this analysis (2). Given the rising incidence of breast cancer over the past four decades, most recently increasing by 0.5% annually from 2010 to 2019, and declining breast cancer mortality (3), we face a growing population of long-term survivors who may continue to experience symptoms from their treatment for many years.

Menopausal symptoms may be triggered in this population by a variety of reasons, including 1) abrupt discontinuation of hormone replacement therapy (HRT) at the time of diagnosis of breast cancer, 2) use of estrogen blockers as a component of breast cancer treatment protocols, and 3) premature menopause in younger women resulting from anti-cancer therapies. There have been a growing number of premenopausal women diagnosed with breast cancer, with more than 12,000 women under the age of 40 years diagnosed with breast cancer annually in the United States (4). Younger women may experience more abrupt and more persistent menopausal symptoms that affect many dimensions of quality of life, and this may lead to early discontinuation or non-initiation of cancer-directed therapies, putting them at an increased risk of cancer recurrence (5, 6).

This chapter will explore the management of vasomotor and genitourinary symptoms in patients diagnosed with breast cancer. We have included in our manuscript references to studies that addressed naturally occurring menopause in women unaffected by breast cancer, as well as women with breast cancer who experienced treatment-induced menopause. The available data suggest that the cause of menopause, whether natural or induced by treatment, has no impact on the efficacy of symptom interventions. Furthermore, there is no way of anticipating what will work best for any given patient, making it imperative to share decision-making and provide steady

DOI: 10.1201/9781032631028-8

follow-up to encourage adherence to breast cancer-directed treatment and to provide guidance for the management of bothersome adverse effects caused by such treatments.

Vasomotor Symptoms

Vasomotor symptoms, which include hot flashes and night sweats, are experienced by most women with breast cancer (7). Menopausal symptoms, including vasomotor symptoms, have been described since at least the nineteenth century, particularly due to the social construction of womanhood and the emphasis on femininity during the time period. In the 1920s, the isolation of estrogen led to hormonal preparations to treat menopausal symptoms, with research since then focusing on risks and benefits of such therapy. In addition, focus has shifted to identify alternative non-hormonal drug therapy, as well as non-pharmacologic therapies to treat vasomotor symptoms (8).

Such symptoms arise in women who received therapies that precipitate a decline in naturally circulating estrogen, either through ovarian failure or estrogen blockade. Suppression of endogenous estrogen levels leads to an imbalance in serotonin concentrations and ultimately disruptions in thermoregulation. While we know this is a common clinical occurrence, it is difficult to ascertain precisely the prevalence and severity of vasomotor symptoms, to a large degree due to underreporting of symptoms. Hot flashes and night sweats may be described in a variety of ways, which make the characterization and grading of symptoms quite challenging. Narrative and qualitative studies provide a better depiction of the patient experience with hot flashes; such data has been used to construct standard definitions of hot flash severity, which have now been incorporated into hot flash scoring systems (9). In clinical trials, the reported incidence of vasomotor symptoms is often about 20–40% lower than in population-based surveys, which identify these symptoms in up to 80% of women (1, 10–12). Studies conducted to assess the reasons and barriers to seeking help with menopausal symptoms have shown that lack of knowledge of the full range of symptoms, stigma, and the belief that such is a normal part of aging, all contribute to underreporting and undertreatment. In addition, women may feel that their symptoms are dismissed by healthcare professionals, and thus they may be reluctant to report or engage in a constructive dialogue with the goal of mitigating unpleasant and distressing symptoms (13).

Management of vasomotor symptoms may include hormonal interventions, non-hormonal drug therapies, and non-pharmacologic therapies.

Non-Estrogenic Pharmacologic Therapies

In patients with naturally driven menopause symptoms, without a current diagnosis or history of breast cancer, hormone replacement therapy (HRT) is a mainstay of treatment. HRT can decrease hot flash severity and frequency by up to 75% (14). The North American Menopause Society 2022 guidelines provide a Level III recommendation, based primarily on consensus and expert opinion, stating systemic hormone therapy is generally not advised for survivors of breast cancer, although it can be considered in patients with severe vasomotor symptoms that are unresponsive. They recommend shared decision making alongside their oncologist, with discussion regarding possible risks (15). A recent meta-analysis conducted to evaluate the safety of HRT on risk of disease recurrence in breast cancer patients found the use of HRT was associated with poor prognostic effect in breast cancer survivors, especially those with hormone receptor-positive disease (16). The current guideline evaluation of the frequency and severity of vasomotor

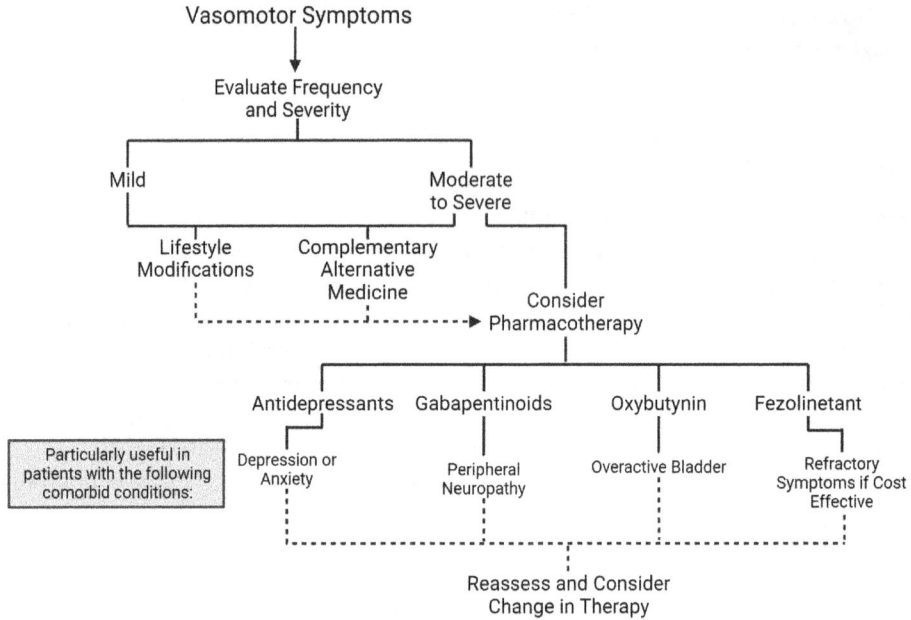

Figure 8.1   An algorithm for management of vasomotor symptoms.

symptoms, as well as identifying comorbid conditions which may benefit from individual treatment options, is a possible pathway to appropriate management of vasomotor symptoms, as described in Figure 8.1.

Antidepressants

The use of antidepressants in the management the of vasomotor symptoms of menopause dates back to 1998, when a pilot study of the serotonin and norepinephrine reuptake inhibitor (SNRI) venlafaxine reported that treatment with low dose venlafaxine (12.5 mg twice daily) for four weeks reduced hot flash scores by 55% in women with a history of breast cancer and men receiving androgen deprivation therapy (17). The mechanism of thermoregulation of both SNRIs and selective serotonin reuptake inhibitors (SSRIs) is complex, involving serotonin's effects on the primary site of thermoregulation, the anterior hypothalamus, and also 5-HT receptors located throughout the peripheral vasomotor and nervous systems (18). Following the pilot study, a placebo-controlled trial evaluated the efficacy of venlafaxine at three doses (37.5 mg, 75mg, and 150 mg daily) versus placebo (19). While all three doses reduced hot flashes, venlafaxine at a dose of 75 mg daily was the best dose to balance efficacy and reduce potential side effects, such as nausea, constipation, and dry mouth. Additional studies conducted examined the effect of desvenlafaxine, an active metabolite of venlafaxine. The two medications have similar side effect profiles, but desvenlafaxine has fewer drug-drug interactions (20). Studies have shown that there is a similar decrease in vasomotor symptoms among venlafaxine and desvenlafaxine (21, 22).

Given the efficacy of SNRIs to manage vasomotor symptoms, research gained traction in evaluating SSRIs for a similar effect, since they produce fewer anticholinergic side effects. Paroxetine, the only FDA-approved antidepressant for the management of vasomotor symptoms, was evaluated in a double blind, placebo-controlled study in 2003 comparing two doses of paroxetine (12.5 mg daily and 25 mg daily) versus a placebo control, over a six-week treatment period. Both paroxetine 12.5 mg daily and 25 mg daily decreased hot flash frequency by 62% and 64%, respectively, compared to a 37% reduction in the placebo group (23). It must also be mentioned that paroxetine is a potent inhibitor of cytochrome P450 2D6, which is the cytochrome system that converts tamoxifen to its active metabolite, theoretically reducing tamoxifen's efficacy. Thus, paroxetine is not the preferred choice for patients who are concurrently receiving tamoxifen therapy, particularly when there are additional antidepressants that may be selected prior, or alternative options as detailed next (24, 25).

Additional SSRIs with improvement in hot flash frequency or severity include both citalopram and escitalopram. Citalopram was evaluated in a phase III trial comparing 10 mg, 20 mg, and 30 mg daily. All three doses improved hot flash scores to a similar degree over a six-week period (50%), but the 20 mg arm noted lower unfavorable impacts of hot flashes on work, sleep, mood, concentration, and quality of life (26). It is currently recommended to start at 10 mg daily and up-titrate as tolerated to the goal dose of 20 mg. In addition, citalopram has been studied in patients who did not have improvement on venlafaxine. Citalopram improved hot flash scores by over 50% after four weeks of treatment (27). This highlights the value in transitioning to a different antidepressant if the first does not provide the desired effect. A prospective randomized controlled trial to evaluate escitalopram versus placebo demonstrated that escitalopram induced at least a 50% reduction of hot flashes in 55% of women who received the trial medication, as compared to 36% in placebo; further, upon discontinuation patients experienced increased hot flashes (28). Tolerability was similarly good in the treatment group, as compared to placebo.

It is important to note that not all SSRIs are equal in their efficacy to manage vasomotor symptoms. For example, fluoxetine, while shown to slightly improve hot flash scores, had only a modest effect size, and when compared with other SSRIs, was less likely to improve hot flashes (29–31). In addition, sertraline has not consistently shown significant difference in decreasing vasomotor symptoms, when compared to placebo (32, 33).

Patients who experience vasomotor symptoms and depression or dysthymia are the ideal patient population to preferentially use SSRIs and SNRIs. When discussing the use of antidepressants for patients with vasomotor symptoms, it is important to highlight the time to effect and dose differences, as compared to their treatment in depression. For most SSRIs and SNRIs, the effect on vasomotor symptoms is quicker than the time each takes to affect mood, and often lower doses produce an effect.

Gabapentinoids

In 2000, a report indicated that gabapentin could be a potential adjunct to relieve vasomotor symptoms. The report assessed six patients who received gabapentin for other indications around the time of hot flashes and, in each patient, was associated with a decrease in their vasomotor symptoms (34). In 2005, a randomized controlled trial in women with breast cancer aimed to study differing doses of gabapentin versus placebo, regarding effects on hot flashes. It revealed that a daily dose of 900 mg (300 mg three times daily) reduced both hot flash frequency and severity, by almost 50% (35). It is hypothesized that during menopause, the number and function of glutamatergic and GABAergic neurons in the hypothalamus changes, thus disrupting the thermoregulatory center. Thus, it is thought that gabapentin lessens the activity in this part of the brain, thereby reducing the number and severity of hot flashes women experience.

Pregabalin, which has a similar mechanism of action as gabapentin, was then studied given its less frequent dosing schedule. A 2010 study reported on the use of pregabalin at 75 mg twice daily versus 150 mg twice daily versus placebo and their effect on hot flash score, which was calculated using self-reported severity and frequency of hot flashes each week. Pregabalin at both 75 mg twice daily and 150 mg twice daily had a significant impact on the hot flash score, with a reduction by 65% and 71%, respectively. Some toxicities were apparent for the pregabalin arms, particularly in the higher dose, including dizziness and cognitive troubles. While this was the case, 60% of participants still found the treatment arm to be beneficial and were able to manage the side effects (36). There is a discrepancy in cost between pregabalin and gabapentin, which may impact patients' ability to access the more expensive pregabalin.

Fezolinetant

Fezolinetant is the newest medication used for the treatment of vasomotor symptoms. It is an orally active selective neurokinin-3 receptor antagonist, which plays a role in the brain's regulation of body temperature. The effectiveness of fezolinetant was demonstrated in two phase III placebo-controlled clinical trials. In both trials, patients were randomized to fezolinetant versus placebo for the first 12 weeks and then transitioned to a 40-week active treatment extension to evaluate safety (37–39). Compared with placebo, fezolinetant at both 30 mg and 40 mg significantly reduced the frequency and severity of vasomotor symptoms at week 4 and maintained this benefit over 52 weeks. The most common side effects included transient liver enzyme elevations (asymptomatic and resolved on treatment or after discontinuation), abdominal pain, and diarrhea.

The largest barrier to the use of fezolinetant is patient access due to cost. The new medication has a list price of $6,600 per year, or $550 per month. While there are patient assistance programs in the US, they have an annual cap of $1,300, and these programs are prohibited in both Medicare and Medicaid, the federal government's provided insurance for elderly patients and state-run insurance program for low-income patients, respectively. The Institute for Clinical and Economic Review (ICER) conducted a cost-effectiveness analysis comparing fezolinetant to hormone replacement therapy and suggested it would be cost-effective if priced at $2,000 annually. In addition, they noted substantial heterogeneity in benefits depending on patient characteristics, including race, ethnicity, BMI, and age (40). An additional study identified patients from five randomized clinical trials, and found that fezolinetant significantly lowered vasomotor symptom frequency and improved menopause-specific quality of life. It was also associated with improvement in sleep quality (41). While the research on fezolinetant and its FDA approval provide an alternative option for non-hormonal management of vasomotor symptoms, additional work is required to allow for widespread access for many patients. Additional research is needed to further understand any potential drug-drug interactions with anticancer therapies.

Oxybutynin

Oxybutynin, an anticholinergic medication used in the treatment of overactive bladder, has multiple anticholinergic effects, including decreased sweating. In 2016, a randomized controlled trial showed that, at a dose of 15 mg daily, oxybutynin resulted in reductions in frequency and severity of hot flashes, but this dose was associated with excessive toxicity and treatment discontinuation (42). In 2020, a randomized controlled trial, in women with and without breast cancer, evaluated lower doses of oxybutynin, 2.5 mg daily and 5 mg daily, regarding the drug's effect on hot flashes, as well as examining side effect severity. Patients on both oxybutynin doses reported reductions in hot flash severity and frequency, and an improvement in a hot flash-related daily interference scale. There were more reported side effects in both oxybutynin arms, including dry mouth and difficulty urinating, but these were reported as grade 1 or 2 side effects, and there was no difference in study discontinuation due to these side effects (43). A confirmatory study that evaluated this drug in men with vasomotor symptoms has completed its accrual goal and should be reported in the near future.

Clonidine

Clonidine is an alpha-adrenergic agent often used for migraine prevention and hypertension. It is hypothesized to affect both hyperhidrosis and hot flashes due to its role mitigating sympathetic stimulation in both conditions. Research into the clinical utility of clonidine is mixed, particularly when compared with other standard therapies. For example, one study showed that venlafaxine more effectively reduces the frequency and severity of hot flashes (44). In another study, venlafaxine improved hot flash frequency and severity faster (4 weeks), but after 12 weeks, there was no difference between venlafaxine and clonidine (45). While the evidence is mixed, clonidine may cause hypotension in some patients. It is thus less frequently used, as compared with other more familiar and tolerable agents.

Progesterone Analogs

Progesterone analogs, including oral megestrol acetate and intramuscular depot medroxyprogesterone acetate (DMPA), are very effective in controlling hot flashes, but their safety when used in women with breast cancer remains to be tested. In 1994, a double blind randomized controlled trial assessed the use of megestrol acetate for the prevention of hot flashes in women during menopause and men who had undergone androgen-deprivation therapy for prostate cancer. Those receiving megestrol acetate had a reduction in their hot flash number by 85%, as compared with 21% in the placebo group (46). Intramuscular DMPA has similar efficacy data and was shown to have significantly improved maintenance of response after 24 weeks as compared with the megestrol group. In addition, its less frequent administration may be preferred for some patients (47). While progesterone analog use in breast cancer patients has often been avoided due to toxicity concerns, an epidemiologic study supported that intramuscular medroxyprogesterone acetate did not increase the risk of recurrent breast cancer (48).

In addition, while the use of combined estrogen and progesterone has been associated with increased risk of venous thromboembolism, there is mixed data on this risk in progesterone only. The US Food and Drug Administration labeling implicates a risk of thrombosis with the use of DMPA, although this risk has not been observed in the limited amount of epidemiologic data. A case-control study conducted by the World Health Organization reported no evidence for an increased risk of stroke, myocardial infarction, or venous thromboembolism with progestin contraceptives, but the power was limited to assess risk of DMPA specifically (49). The possible risk of venous thromboembolism in progesterone only analogs should be discussed with breast cancer patients given their increased risk of thromboembolism due to malignancy.

Non-Pharmacologic Therapies

In addition to pharmacologic measures, patients express interest in seeking non-pharmacologic therapies; these include lifestyle and integrative therapies, oral supplements, and behavioral interventions. Complementary and alternative medicine (CAM) is a term used to describe medical therapies that fall beyond the scope of conventional medical practice, but may be used alongside it in the treatment of illness and disease. In fact, over 51% of menopausal women use CAM, and more than 60% perceive it to be effective for menopausal symptoms (50). Effective communication with patients regarding their beliefs and practices provides value in identifying possible CAM therapies that may be of interest to specific individuals (51).

This section will provide a brief overview of oral supplements and additional therapy measures, ranging from cognitive behavioral therapy to stellate ganglion block.

Lifestyle Measures

The evidence behind lifestyle and behavioral measures to manage vasomotor symptoms is limited and mixed, although these measures can help improve wellbeing and may help women tolerate symptoms, with little risk of adverse effects. Patients are encouraged to promote cooling through different environmental measures, because slight changes in core body temperature elevations can trigger vasomotor symptoms (52–55). These techniques include dressing in layers, use of fans, drinking cool liquids, and cooling techniques at bedtime, including using cold packs under a pillow. An interesting means of doing so came from a story of a woman in San Francisco who noted that, in the winter, she would get in her car, put on her seatbelt, and then put her coat on backwards, so it could be easily shed when she was driving. Additionally, it is recommended that women attempt to identify and avoid possible triggers of vasomotor symptoms. Common triggers include spicy foods, tobacco use, alcohol, and caffeine. There is also evidence that weight gain may increase severity of vasomotor symptoms. Breast cancer survivors with a post-diagnosis weight gain had a greater risk of reporting hot flashes. In a study of 40 overweight or obese women, a 10% weight loss resulted in significant improvement in hot flashes (56). Providing education, time, and lifestyle modifications are reasonable options to provide anticipatory guidance to patients with mild vasomotor symptoms. For patients with moderate to severe symptoms, which affect many aspects of daily life and may inhibit adherence to disease directed treatment, early initiation of pharmacologic measures should be considered.

Oral Supplements

Phytoestrogens are nonsteroidal plant-derived compounds, with similar properties to estrogen. There are two major classes of phytoestrogens: isoflavones (soy) and lignans (flaxseed, whole grain, legumes). Depending on the level of endogenous estrogen in the body, phytoestrogens can have estrogenic properties (low endogenous levels) or anti-estrogenic properties (high endogenous levels). A meta-analysis and systematic review conducted in 2015 examined the efficacy of phytoestrogens to treat menopausal symptoms. The review identified 15 randomized controlled trials, and in the 10 studies that reported on hot flash data, phytoestrogens resulted in a significant reduction in hot flash frequency when compared to placebo without a significant side effect profile (57). Nonetheless, the data regarding phytoestrogens is quite heterogenous with regards to exact compound, formulation, and dose, and thus it is difficult to draw definitive conclusions.

Vitamin E is a fat-soluble vitamin with anti-inflammatory properties, thought to act as an antioxidant in the body. Vitamin E supplementation is often very well tolerated, but there is insufficient empirical evidence to decide on its effectiveness at this time. One crossover trial of 120 women receiving 800 IU of vitamin E followed by placebo reported a statistically significant decrease of one hot flash per day with vitamin E, but this result was not clinically significant (58). In another crossover trial of 50 women receiving 500 IU of vitamin E versus placebo, patients had a reduction in two hot flashes per day and reduced hot flash severity (59). Another randomized placebo-controlled trial provided negative results (58). In aggregate, results suggest that vitamin E may be slightly better than placebo; however, it is unlikely to be as effective as the pharmacologic therapies outlined earlier.

Black cohosh is a perennial herb which has been used for many years in European and Asian countries. The specific mechanism in reducing hot flashes is not fully understood but may be attributed to binding and modulation of central nervous system receptors, including serotonin, dopamine, and GABA (60, 61). The efficacy of black cohosh is still debated, decades after it was adopted by women seeking relief from vasomotor symptoms. There have been many recent meta-analyses conducted to evaluate, with one in 2023 which revealed significant improvement in menopausal symptoms and hot flashes as compared to placebo (62). Regardless of the debated efficacy, there have been over 30 cases of hepatotoxicity, and caution is recommended (63).

Behavioral Therapies, Acupuncture, Hypnosis, and Stellate Ganglion Block

When performed by trained specialists, acupuncture, cognitive behavior therapy, hypnosis, and stellate ganglion blocks can provide additional benefit, and be potentially additive to pharmacologic treatment. For example, two multicenter RCTs have reported that acupuncture improves hot flashes when compared to usual or enhanced self-care (64, 65). Current research is being conducted to identify clinical and genomic identifiers that may predict the responsiveness to acupuncture treatment.

In addition, both cognitive behavioral therapy and hypnosis have been studied as mind-body approaches with effect on hot flash symptoms. In a randomized controlled trial of 187 postmenopausal women reporting at least seven hot flashes per day, the use of five weekly sessions of hypnosis saw a mean reduction of hot flash frequency by 74% (66). In another randomized trial, the MENOS 1 trial, which compared usual care alone and usual care with six weeks of cognitive behavioral therapy, the group with cognitive behavioral therapy had a significant reduction in the burden of hot flashes, with the result sustained after 26 weeks (67). The amount of evidence to support either intervention is small but promising and highlights a need for additional research (68).

A final intervention to highlight is the use of a stellate ganglion block. Stellate ganglion blocks involve injection of a local anesthetic to the stellate ganglion. When performed by experienced providers, blocks are very well tolerated with limited risk of serious complications. Studies have shown that stellate ganglion blocks decreased the frequency of moderate to very severe hot flashes by 52% (69).

Vasomotor Symptoms in Men on Hormonal Therapy

It is important to identify and manage vasomotor symptoms in men. While the management strategies are similar to those in women, it is reported that men are less likely to report vasomotor symptoms than women (70). Hot flashes can occur in healthy aging men, men with breast cancer treated with endocrine therapy, and men with prostate cancer treated with hormone deprivation therapy. The incidence of breast cancer in men is increasing over the last 10 years (71). Furthermore, prostate cancer is the most common form of cancer in men, with approximately 288,030 new cancer cases diagnosed in 2023 in the United States (72). The incidence of hot flashes in men with breast cancer remains understudied. In men with prostate cancer treated with orchiectomy, 58–76% reported hot flashes and, in those treated with GnRH analogues, a medical form of castration, 75% experienced hot flashes (73, 74). Prior studies have shown that men who do not take a treatment for hot flashes report unchanged hot flash severity and frequency over time, highlighting a long persistence of hot flashes after treatment. After men have completed anti-cancer therapies, it is common for total testosterone to remain at castrate levels, particularly in older men. Given the increasing incidence of breast cancer in men, high number of prostate cancer cases in men, and large number of men with prostate cancer and breast cancer experiencing hot flashes, it is important to direct attention to this symptom complex in male cancer survivors.

One patient, currently receiving androgen deprivation therapy for prostate cancer, recounts the impact hot flashes have on his quality of life. "The sudden onset of the hot flashes interferes with my daily life, and can often occur multiple times a day. I worry about being in a meeting at work, or out to dinner with friends, and not being able to manage my symptoms. I am often torn between the positive impact of therapy and its effect on my cancer, and the difficult to manage side effects, which detrimentally impact my day to day life" (Interview with a person who requested anonymity, personal communication, March 16, 2025).

Overall Approach to Management of Vasomotor Symptoms

The overall approach to the management of vasomotor symptoms should begin with effective communication with all individuals who are diagnosed with breast cancer to identify and understand symptom burden and effect on quality of life. Education should be provided on the natural history of hot flashes, lifestyle measures, and avoidance of possible triggers. Close follow-up with these patients and subsequent inquiry into vasomotor symptoms should be performed. Following education and lifestyle measures, the preferred options for non-estrogenic medication therapy include antidepressants, such as venlafaxine, desvenlafaxine, citalopram, escitalopram, and paroxetine, as well as pregabalin, gabapentin, oxybutynin, and fezolinetant. Initial medical management should take into consideration the individual patient's comorbidities, possible drug-drug interactions, and patient preferences of possible medication side effects (see Table 8.1). If one therapy is ineffective, it is reasonable to try another, even within drug classes. In addition to medical management, the use of complementary and integrative therapies can be helpful and may be preferred by the patient.

Table 8.1A   Interventions and Adverse Effects

Intervention	Common Adverse Effects	Serious (Rare) Adverse Effects
Antidepressants	Weight gain Sexual dysfunction Diarrhea Hypertension Fatigue	Serotonin syndrome SIADH
Gabapentinoids	Weight gain Drowsiness Fatigue	CNS/respiratory depression Angioedema
Oxybutynin	Dry mouth Constipation Urinary retention	Agitated delirium Narrow-angle glaucoma
Progesterone analogs	Weight gain Depression Abdominal pain Mastalgia Myalgia	Possible breast cancer risk Possible VTE risk

Table 8.1B   Properties of and Considerations with Medications

Agent	Recommended Starting Dose	Recommended Target Dose	Considerations
Citalopram	10 mg daily	20 mg daily	First-line agent for most patients
Escitalopram	10 mg daily	20 mg daily	First-line agent for most patients
Paroxetine	10 mg daily	10 mg daily	Only FDA-approved agent Avoid in patients taking tamoxifen due to CYP2D6 blockade
Venlafaxine	37.5 mg daily	75 mg daily	Careful dose escalation and tapering due to acute toxicity and withdrawal
Desvenlafaxine	50 mg daily	100–150 mg daily	Similar to venlafaxine, there may be cost differences
Gabapentin	300 mg once daily at bedtime	300 mg three times a day	Three times a day dosing schedule
Pregabalin	50 mg once daily at bedtime	75 mg twice daily	More convenient dosing schedule than gabapentin, less studied
Oxybutynin	2.5 mg twice daily	5 mg twice daily	Can cause adverse events particularly in elderly
Fezolinetant	45 mg daily	45 mg daily	May be cost prohibitive, perform liver function tests prior to initiation

Genitourinary Symptoms

The genitourinary syndrome of menopause (GSM) encompasses various symptoms caused by changes of the vulva, vagina, and lower urinary tract that are associated with decreased estrogen levels. The GSM may be characterized by genital dryness, irritation, burning, sexual symptoms (lack of lubrication, discomfort or pain), and urinary symptoms (urgency, dysuria, recurrent urinary tract infections) (75). In large cohort studies, 45% to 63% of postmenopausal women reported symptoms consistent with GSM, the most common being vaginal dryness (76). In addition, other studies reported that women with sexual dysfunction, such as lack of desire, arousal difficulties, and orgasmic difficulties, found that vaginal dryness was an important associated factor (77).

Although there are safe and effective therapies for GSM, fewer than 40% of women receive treatment due to both clinician and patient reluctance to discuss and evaluate these symptoms (78). Screening tools have been created to assess a patient's interest in discussing topics and can be used to further guide conversations about GSMs and their impact on a patient's overall quality of life. The most common assessment tools include the visual analog scale (VAS), the vaginal health index (VHI), and the female sexual function index (FSFI) patient-reported outcomes measure (PROM) (79). FSFI, for example, is a subjective measure to assess six domains of sexuality, including lubrication, orgasm, satisfaction, desire, arousal, and pain. Alternatively, the VHI is a clinical medical evaluation, evaluating vaginal elasticity, fluid volume, epithelial integrity, and moisture.

Local Hormonal Therapy

Local hormonal therapy for GSM includes local estrogen therapy in the form of vaginal tablets, inserts, creams, rings, and vaginal dehydroepiandrosterone (DHEA). For local estrogen therapy, use of these formulations in breast cancer survivors may be met with reluctance due to their unclear long-term safety and concerns for systemic absorption. Despite the high prevalence of GSM, in a retrospective study of 176,012 patients on hormone therapy for breast cancer, only 3% of women receiving tamoxifen or an aromatase inhibitor were also filling prescriptions for topical estrogen (80). In addition, a study conducted to survey breast surgeons, urogynecologists, and gynecologists revealed that many felt comfortable prescribing topical estrogen to patients with a history of ER-negative breast cancer or patients who had completed endocrine therapy but were less comfortable using topical estrogen for those who were actively receiving endocrine therapy (81).

The unclear long-term safety and its infrequent utilization are due in part to the uncertainty regarding the systemic absorption of local estrogen therapy. Studies have shown that there is acute systemic absorption of almost all vaginal estrogen preparations, but the question is if this absorption is enough to stimulate breast cancer proliferation (82). There are few large studies that have examined the long-term safety of these formulations in patients with ER-positive breast cancer. Currently, the American College of Obstetricians and Gynecologists and the North American Menopause Society recommend reserving topical estrogen therapies for those who have failed nonhormonal therapies (83, 84). In addition, they can be considered in patients with cancers that are not driven by estrogen, those with low-grade disease, or those with a remote history of breast cancer with a low risk of recurrence.

Vaginal DHEA is a precursor hormone that is aromatized to form an estrogenic compound. Studies have shown mixed efficacy, with one study comparing 3.25 mg/day DHEA, 6.5 mg/day DHEA, and a plain moisturizer which revealed that all arms had improvement in vaginal dryness, but neither dose of DHEA was superior to the plain moisturizer. There was an increase in systemic concentrations of sex hormones, but these levels differed by concomitant endocrine therapy use. There was no increase in estrogen concentration that was observed in women who were on an aromatase inhibitor (85). Additional research is needed to further understand the efficacy and safety profile of vaginal DHEA.

Non-Estrogenic Therapy

Nonhormonal-based treatments are considered first-line therapy for GSM in patients with a history of estrogen-dependent breast cancer, particularly for the management of vaginal dryness, vaginal atrophy, and dyspareunia. Many treatments have shown to be effective, including lubricants, moisturizers, vaginal suppositories, and aqueous lidocaine.

Plain vaginal moisturizers, such as Replens, can be used to hydrate the vaginal mucosa. These products compare favorably to vaginal estrogen therapy (86, 87). In addition, vaginal gels containing polyacrylic acid or hyaluronic acid also have a moisturizing component. In a small trial of women taking tamoxifen, patients who were randomized to polyacrylic acid reported a decrease in sexual dysfunction from 96% to 24% (88). When used three to five times per week, hyaluronic acid has been shown to improve sexual function among breast cancer survivors (89, 90).

Compared to moisturizers, the function of vaginal lubricants is to decrease friction. There are multiple formulations of lubricants, including polycarbophil-, silicone-, and water-based lubricants. Patients should review a product's package insert prior to use with barrier methods, since certain lubricants should not be used with condoms. When compared with a water-based lubricant, a polycarbophil-based lubricant was superior in reducing dyspareunia (91). In addition, silicone-based lubricants were found to provide improved symptomatic relief, when compared to water-based lubricant (92).

In addition, vitamin D and E suppositories have been shown to cause a decrease in vaginal pH, with subsequent improvement in vaginal atrophy symptoms (93). Topical lidocaine may also be effective for patients who experience introital pain. In a double-blind trial of breast cancer survivors with penetrative introital pain, the use of 4% aqueous lidocaine applied prior to vaginal intercourse was associated with reduction in dyspareunia by 88% (94).

Vaginal Laser Therapy

Vaginal laser therapy can be an alternative option, particularly in patients in whom non-hormonal therapy is not effective and there is a relative contraindication to hormonal therapy. Vaginal CO_2 laser therapy remodels vaginal tissue by activation of fibroblasts, collagen production, and neovascularization (95). Current evidence behind vaginal laser therapy is promising with regards to its ability to reduce vaginal symptoms, including a non-randomized prospective observational trial of 50 breast cancer survivors, which showed improvement in the severity of dyspareunia and in the vaginal health index, which reflects vaginal elasticity, fluid volume, pH, epithelial integrity, and moisture (96). In addition, there is a systematic review evaluating ten observational studies of GSM symptoms in breast cancer patients before and after vaginal laser therapy, which showed improvement in vaginal health index and visual analog scale in the short term, with additional research needed to evaluate long-term benefit (97). There is also a recent retrospective study of 82 breast cancer survivors with vaginal atrophy in spite of non-estrogenic therapy, who had improvement in all symptoms (98). Evidence is limited due to small sample size, short follow-up, inconsistent laser dose, and lack of a placebo control.

There are currently multiple ongoing studies exploring the effect of vaginal laser therapy on GSM (97). One study is composed of three separate sub-studies, including a dose response study, a randomized controlled trial, and a follow-up study. The primary endpoint is vaginal dryness, but additional secondary endpoints are being evaluated, including vaginal pain, itching, soreness, urinary symptoms, sexual function, change in vaginal histology (punch biopsy), change in vaginal and urine microbiota, and change in vaginal pH (99). Another ongoing study is a phase III randomized study comparing fractional CO_2 laser treatments with sham laser treatments, with crossover occurring in the sham laser treatment after three sessions (NCT05379153). The primary outcome will evaluate patient-reported symptoms with a vaginal assessment scale, and the secondary outcome is objective findings of atrophy on examination. Patients will be followed for 24 months to allow for long-term follow-up. Cost may be a significant barrier to accessing vaginal laser therapy, since it is often not covered by insurance in the US and can be prohibitively expensive.

Conclusion

Menopausal symptoms, while often underreported, remain important targets for intervention to improve health related quality of life among breast cancer survivors. Evidence-based and evidence-informed interventions have been shown to mitigate vasomotor symptoms, improve sleep, and improve or restore genitourinary and sexual health. Finding the right approach depends on many factors including symptom frequency and severity, while the decision to intervene ultimately rests with the patient. We recommend that clinicians caring for breast cancer survivors and people with other cancers who also experience distressing menopausal symptoms engage in frank conversations and provide guidance and referrals as needed, with the goal of optimizing their health after cancer.

References

1. Harris PF et al. Prevalence and treatment of menopausal symptoms among breast cancer survivors. J Pain Symptom Manage. 2002;23(6):501–9.
2. Hickey M et al. Managing menopause after cancer. Lancet. 2024;403(10430):984–96.
3. Giaquinto AN et al. Breast cancer statistics, 2022. CA Cancer J Clin. 2022;72(6):524–41.
4. Guo F et al. Trends in breast cancer mortality by stage at diagnosis among young women in the United States. Cancer. 2018;124(17):3500–9.
5. Bernhard J et al. Patient-reported outcomes with adjuvant exemestane versus tamoxifen in premenopausal women with early breast cancer undergoing ovarian suppression (TEXT and SOFT): A combined analysis of two phase 3 randomised trials. Lancet Oncol. 2015;16(7):848–58.
6. Perrone G et al. Menopausal symptoms after the discontinuation of long-term hormone replacement therapy in women under 60: A 3-year follow-up. Gynecol Obstet Invest. 2013;76(1):38–43.
7. Gupta P et al. Menopausal symptoms in women treated for breast cancer: The prevalence and severity of symptoms and their perceived effects on quality of life. Climacteric. 2006;9(1):49–58.
8. Singh A et al. A historical perspective on menopause and menopausal age. Bull Indian Inst Hist Med Hyderabad. 2002;32(2):121–35.
9. Finck G et al. Definitions of hot flashes in breast cancer survivors. J Pain Symptom Manag. 1998;16(5):327–33.
10. Chang HY et al. Hot flashes in breast cancer survivors: Frequency, severity and impact. Breast. 2016;27:116–21.
11. Howell A et al. Results of the ATAC (Arimidex, Tamoxifen, Alone or in Combination) trial after completion of 5 years' adjuvant treatment for breast cancer. Lancet. 2005;365(9453):60–2.
12. Kligman L, Younus J. Management of hot flashes in women with breast cancer. Curr Oncol. 2010;17(1):81–6.
13. Barber K, Charles A. Barriers to accessing effective treatment and support for menopausal symptoms: A qualitative study capturing the behaviours, beliefs and experiences of key stakeholders. Patient Prefer Adherence. 2023;17:2971–80.
14. Maclennan AH et al. Oral oestrogen and combined oestrogen/progestogen therapy versus placebo for hot flushes. Cochrane Database Syst Rev. 2004;2004(4):CD002978.
15. Advisory P. The 2022 hormone therapy position statement of the North American Menopause Society. Menopause. 2022;29(7):767–94.
16. Poggio F et al. Safety of systemic hormone replacement therapy in breast cancer survivors: A systematic review and meta-analysis. Breast Cancer Res Treat. 2022;191(2):269–75.
17. Loprinzi CL et al. Pilot evaluation of venlafaxine hydrochloride for the therapy of hot flashes in cancer survivors. J Clin Oncol. 1998;16(7):2377–81.
18. Schwartz PJ et al. Serotonin and thermoregulation: Physiologic and pharmacologic aspects of control revealed by intravenous m-CPP in normal human subjects. Neuropsychopharmacol. 1995;13(2):105–15.
19. Loprinzi CL et al. Venlafaxine in management of hot flashes in survivors of breast cancer: A randomised controlled trial. Lancet. 2000;356(9247):2059–63.
20. Preskorn SH et al. Effect of desvenlafaxine on the cytochrome P450 2D6 enzyme system. J Psychiatr Pract. 2008;14(6):368–78.
21. Archer DF et al. Desvenlafaxine for the treatment of vasomotor symptoms associated with menopause: A double-blind, randomized, placebo-controlled trial of efficacy and safety. Am J Obstet Gynecol. 2009;200(3):238e1–10.
22. Pinkerton JV et al. Desvenlafaxine compared with placebo for treatment of menopausal vasomotor symptoms: A 12-week, multicenter, parallel-group, randomized, double-blind, placebo-controlled efficacy trial. Menopause. 2013;20(1):28–37.
23. Stearns V et al. Paroxetine controlled release in the treatment of menopausal hot flashes: A randomized controlled trial. JAMA. 2003;289(21):2827–34.
24. Kelly CM et al. Selective serotonin reuptake inhibitors and breast cancer mortality in women receiving tamoxifen: A population based cohort study. BMJ. 2010;340:c693.

25. Stearns V et al. Active tamoxifen metabolite plasma concentrations after coadministration of tamoxifen and the selective serotonin reuptake inhibitor paroxetine. J Natl Cancer Inst. 2003;95(23):1758–64.
26. Barton DL et al. Phase III, placebo-controlled trial of three doses of citalopram for the treatment of hot flashes: NCCTG trial N05C9. J Clin Oncol. 2010;28(20):3278–83.
27. Loprinzi CL et al. Pilot evaluation of citalopram for the treatment of hot flashes in women with inadequate benefit from venlafaxine. J Palliat Med. 2005;8(5):24–30.
28. Freeman EW et al. Efficacy of escitalopram for hot flashes in healthy menopausal women: A randomized controlled trial. JAMA. 2011;305(3):267–74.
29. Loprinzi CL et al. Phase III evaluation of fluoxetine for treatment of hot flashes. J Clin Oncol. 2002;20(6):1578–83.
30. Shams T et al. SSRIs for hot flashes: A systematic review and meta-analysis of randomized trials. J Gen Intern Med. 2014;29(1):204–13.
31. Loprinzi CL et al. Newer antidepressants and gabapentin for hot flashes: An individual patient pooled analysis. J Clin Oncol. 2009;27(17):2831–7.
32. Grady D et al. Ineffectiveness of sertraline for treatment of menopausal hot flushes: A randomized controlled trial. Obstet Gynecol. 2007;109(4):823–30.
33. Kerwin JP et al. The variable response of women with menopausal hot flashes when treated with sertraline. Menopause. 2007;14(5):841–5.
34. Guttuso TJ Jr. Gabapentin's effects on hot flashes and hypothermia. Neurology. 2000;54(11):2161–3.
35. Pandya KJ et al. Gabapentin for hot flashes in 420 women with breast cancer: A randomised double-blind placebo-controlled trial. Lancet. 2005;366(9488):818–24.
36. Loprinzi CL et al. Phase III, randomized, double-blind, placebo-controlled evaluation of pregabalin for alleviating hot flashes, N07C1. J Clin Oncol. 2010;28(4):641–7.
37. Johnson KA et al. Efficacy and safety of fezolinetant in moderate to severe vasomotor symptoms associated with menopause: A phase 3 RCT. J Clin Endocrinol Metab. 2023;108(8):1981–97.
38. Neal-Perry G et al. Safety of fezolinetant for vasomotor symptoms associated with menopause: A randomized controlled trial. Obstet Gynecol. 2023;141(4):737–47.
39. Lederman S et al. Fezolinetant for treatment of moderate-to-severe vasomotor symptoms associated with menopause (SKYLIGHT 1): A phase 3 randomised controlled study. Lancet. 2023;401(10382):1091–102.
40. Wright AC et al. The effectiveness and value of fezolinetant for moderate-to-severe vasomotor symptoms associated with menopause: A summary from the Institute for Clinical and Economic Review's Midwest Public Advisory Council. J Manag Care Spec Pharm. 2023;29(6):692–8.
41. Bonga KN et al. Efficacy and safety of fezolinetant for the treatment of menopause-associated vasomotor symptoms: A meta-analysis. Obstet Gynecol. 2024;143(3):393–402.
42. Simon JA et al. Extended-release oxybutynin therapy for vasomotor symptoms in women: A randomized clinical trial. Menopause. 2016;23(11):1214–21.
43. Leon-Ferre RA et al. Oxybutynin vs placebo for hot flashes in women with or without breast cancer: A randomized, double-blind clinical trial (ACCRU SC-1603). JNCI Cancer Spectr. 2020;4(1):pkz088.
44. Loibl S et al. Venlafaxine is superior to clonidine as treatment of hot flashes in breast cancer patients—a double-blind, randomized study. Ann Oncol. 2007;18(4):689–93.
45. Boekhout AH et al. Management of hot flashes in patients who have breast cancer with venlafaxine and clonidine: A randomized, double-blind, placebo-controlled trial. J Clin Oncol. 2011;29(29):3862–8.
46. Loprinzi CL et al. Megestrol acetate for the prevention of hot flashes. N Engl J Med. 1994;331(6):347–52.
47. Bertelli G et al. Intramuscular depot medroxyprogesterone versus oral megestrol for the control of postmenopausal hot flashes in breast cancer patients: A randomized study. Ann Oncol. 2002;13(6):883–8.
48. Ertz-Archambault NM et al. Depomedroxyprogesterone acetate therapy for hot flashes in survivors of breast cancer: No unfavorable impact on recurrence and survival. Support Care Cancer. 2020;28(5):2139–43.
49. World Health Organization Collaborative Study of Cardiovascular Disease and Steroid Hormone Contraception. Cardiovascular disease and use of oral and injectable progestogen-only contraceptives and combined injectable contraceptives. Results of an international, multicenter, case-control study. Contraception. 1998;57(5):315–24.

50. Posadzki P et al. Prevalence of complementary and alternative medicine (CAM) use by menopausal women: A systematic review of surveys. Maturitas. 2013;75(1):34–43.

51. Ma J et al. US women desire greater professional guidance on hormone and alternative therapies for menopause symptom management. Menopause. 2006;13(3):506–16.

52. Nonhormonal management of menopause-associated vasomotor symptoms: 2015 position statement of The North American Menopause Society. Menopause. 2015 Nov;22(11):1155–72. Quiz: 1173–4. doi: 10.1097/GME.0000000000000546. PMID: 26382310.

53. Freedman RR et al. Core body temperature and circadian rhythm of hot flashes in menopausal women. J Clin Endocrinol Metab. 1995;80(8):2354–8.

54. Freedman RR, Woodward S. Core body temperature during menopausal hot flushes. Fertil Steril. 1996;65(6):1141–4.

55. Marshall-McKenna R et al. A randomised trial of the cool pad pillow topper versus standard care for sleep disturbance and hot flushes in women on endocrine therapy for breast cancer. Support Care Cancer. 2016;24(4):1821–9.

56. Caan BJ et al. Effect of postdiagnosis weight change on hot flash status among early-stage breast cancer survivors. J Clin Oncol. 2012;30(13):1492–7.

57. Chen MN et al. Efficacy of phytoestrogens for menopausal symptoms: A meta-analysis and systematic review. Climacteric. 2015;18(2):260–9.

58. Barton DL et al. Prospective evaluation of vitamin E for hot flashes in breast cancer survivors. J Clin Oncol. 1998;16(2):495–500.

59. Ziaei SA et al. The effect of vitamin E on hot flashes in menopausal women. Gynecol Obstet Investig. 2007;64(4):204–7.

60. Powell SL et al. In vitro serotonergic activity of black cohosh and identification of N(omega)-methylserotonin as a potential active constituent. J Agric Food Chem. 2008;56(24):11718–26.

61. Cicek SS et al. Bioactivity-guided isolation of GABA(A) receptor modulating constituents from the rhizomes of Actaea racemosa. J Nat Prod. 2010;73(12):2024–8.

62. Sadahiro R et al. Black cohosh extracts in women with menopausal symptoms: An updated pairwise meta-analysis. Menopause. 2023;30(7):766–73.

63. Mahady GB et al. United States pharmacopeia review of the black cohosh case reports of hepatotoxicity. Menopause. 2008;15(4 Pt 1):628–38.

64. Kim KH et al. Effects of acupuncture on hot flashes in perimenopausal and postmenopausal women—a multicenter randomized clinical trial. Menopause. 2010;17(2):269–80.

65. Lesi G et al. Acupuncture as an integrative approach for the treatment of hot flashes in women with breast cancer: A prospective multicenter randomized controlled trial (AcCliMaT). J Clin Oncol. 2016;34(15):1795–802.

66. Elkins GR et al. Clinical hypnosis in the treatment of postmenopausal hot flashes: A randomized controlled trial. Menopause. 2013;20(3):291–8.

67. Mann E et al. Cognitive behavioral treatment for women who have menopausal symptoms after breast cancer treatment (MENOS 1): A randomised controlled trial. Lancet Oncol. 2012;13(3):309–18.

68. Elkins G et al. Randomized trial of a hypnosis intervention for treatment of hot flashes among breast cancer survivors. J Clin Oncol. 2008;26(31):5022–6.

69. Walega DR et al. Effects of stellate ganglion block on vasomotor symptoms: Findings from a randomized controlled clinical trial in postmenopausal women. Menopause. 2014;21(8):807–14.

70. Eziefula CU et al. "You know I've joined your club . . . I'm the hot flush boy": A qualitative exploration of hot flushes and night sweats in men undergoing androgen deprivation therapy for prostate cancer. Psychooncology. 2013;22(12):823–30.

71. Konduri S et al. Epidemiology of male breast cancer. Breast. 2020;54:8–14.

72. Siegel RL et al. Cancer statistics, 2023. CA Cancer J Clin. 2023;73(1):17–48.

73. Charig CR, Rundle JS. Flushing. Long-term side effect of orchiectomy in treatment of prostatic carcinoma. Urology. 1989;33(3):175–8.

74. Smith JA Jr. Androgen suppression by a gonadotropin releasing hormone analogue in patients with metastatic carcinoma of the prostate. J Urol. 1984;131(6):1110–2.

75. Kim HK et al. The recent review of the genitourinary syndrome of menopause. J Menopausal Med. 2015;21(2):65–71.

76. Nappi RE, Kokot-Kierepa M. Women's voices in the menopause: Results from an international survey on vaginal atrophy. Maturitas. 2010;67(3):233–8.
77. Avis NE et al. Longitudinal changes in sexual functioning as women transition through menopause: Results from the study of Women's Health Across the Nation. Menopause. 2009;16(3):442–52.
78. Cook ED et al. Missing documentation in breast cancer survivors: Genitourinary syndrome of menopause. Menopause. 2017;24(12):1360–4.
79. Mension E et al. Genitourinary syndrome of menopause assessment tools. J Mid-Life Health. 2021;12(2):99–102.
80. Huntley JH et al. Topical estrogen prescription fill rates for women with a history of breast cancer who are taking hormone therapy. Obstet Gynecol. 2018;132(5):1137–42.
81. Richter LA et al. Topical estrogen prescribing patterns for urogenital atrophy among women with breast cancer: Results of a national provider survey. Menopause. 2019;26(7):714–19.
82. Santen RJ. Vaginal administration of estradiol: Effects of dose, preparation and timing on plasma estradiol levels. Climacteric. 2015;18(2):121–34.
83. ACOG committee opinion 659: The use of vaginal estrogen in women with a history of estrogen-dependent breast cancer. Obstet Gynecol. 2016;127(3):e93–6.
84. Faubion SS et al. Management of genitourinary syndrome of menopause in women with or at high risk for breast cancer: Consensus recommendations from The North American Menopause Society and The International Society for the study of Women's Sexual Health. Menopause. 2018;25(6):596–608.
85. Barton DL et al. Systemic and local effects of vaginal dehydroepiandrosterone (DHEA): NCCTG N10C1 (Alliance). Support Care Cancer. 2018;26(4):1335–43.
86. Bygdeman M, Swahn ML. Replens versus dienoestrol cream in the symptomatic treatment of vaginal atrophy in postmenopausal women. Maturitas. 1996;23(3):259–63.
87. Mitchell CM et al. Efficacy of vaginal estradiol or vaginal moisturizer vs placebo for treating postmenopausal vulvovaginal symptoms: A randomized clinical trial. JAMA Intern Med. 2018;178(5):681–90.
88. Juliato PT et al. Can polyacrylic acid treat sexual dysfunction in women with breast cancer receiving tamoxifen? Climacteric. 2017;20(1):62–6.
89. Krychman M, Millheiser LS. Sexual health issues in women with cancer. J Sex Med. 2013; 10(1_suppl):5–15.
90. Carter J et al. A single-arm, prospective trial investigating the effectiveness of a non-hormonal vaginal moisturizer containing hyaluronic acid in postmenopausal cancer survivors. Support Care Cancer. 2021;29(1):311–22.
91. Loprinzi CL et al. Phase III randomized double-blind study to evaluate the efficacy of a polycarbophil-based vaginal moisturizer in women with breast cancer. J Clin Oncol. 1997;15(3):969–73.
92. Hickey M et al. A randomized, double-blind, crossover trial comparing a silicone- versus water-based lubricant for sexual discomfort after breast cancer. Breast Cancer Res Treat. 2016;158(1):79–90.
93. Keshavarzi Z et al. The effect of vitamin D and E vaginal suppositories on tamoxifen-induced vaginal atrophy in women with breast cancer. Support Care Cancer. 2019;27(4):1325–34.
94. Goetsch MF et al. Locating pain in breast cancer survivors experiencing dyspareunia: A randomized controlled trial. Obstet Gynecol. 2014;123(6):1231–6.
95. Sokol ER, Karram MM. Use of a novel fractional CO_2 laser for the treatment of genitourinary syndrome of menopause: 1-year outcomes. Menopause. 2017;24(7):810–4.
96. Pieralli A et al. Fractional CO_2 laser for vulvovaginal atrophy (VVA) dyspareunia relief in breast cancer survivors. Arch Gynecol Obstet. 2016;294(4):841–6.
97. Jha S et al. The impact of vaginal laser treatment for genitourinary syndrome of menopause in breast cancer survivors: A systematic review and meta-analysis. Clin Breast Cancer. 2019 Aug;19(4):e556–62. doi: 10.1016/j.clbc.2019.04.007. Epub 2019 Apr 19. PMID: 31227415.
98. Pagano T et al. Fractional microablative CO_2 laser in breast cancer survivors affected by iatrogenic vulvovaginal atrophy after failure of nonestrogenic local treatments: A retrospective study. Menopause. 2018;25(6):657–62.
99. Jacobsen S et al. Vaginal $CO(2)$ laser therapy for genitourinary syndrome in breast cancer survivors-VagLaser study protocol: A randomized blinded, placebo-controlled trial. BMC Cancer. 2023;23(1):1164.

Chapter 9

Gynecologic Cancers: From Epidemiology to Survivorship

Alexa Steckler, Kang Woo Kim, Don S. Dizon and
Christine A. Duffy

Introduction

The pelvic cancers in women include those that arise in the female reproductive tract, vagina, and vulva. Collectively they compose the gynecologic cancers. While in general they most commonly arise in postmenopausal women, they do arise in women with intact ovarian function who become—or are at heightened risk for—early menopause. In this section we provide an overview of the major gynecologic cancers that may impact women prior to menopause, survivorship following these diagnoses, and specifically, what is known about treatment for menopausal symptoms with an emphasis on oral hormone therapy (HT).

An Overview of the Pelvic Cancers in Women

Endometrial Cancer

Epidemiology

According to the 2020 Global Cancer Report, endometrial cancer ranked second in female gynecologic cancer incidence worldwide, with 417,367 new cases and 97,000 deaths (1). The rise is in part attributed to obesity and physical inactivity, especially in high-income countries, although it tracks with the overall aging of the population (2). In the US, incidence has continued to increase by about 1% per year since the mid-2000s, especially for non-White Americans (Black, Hispanic, and Asian American and Pacific Islander women) (1). While most patients diagnosed with endometrial cancer are postmenopausal (the median age at diagnosis is 60 years), up to 14% of cases occur in premenopausal women, particularly with elevated body mass index (BMI) (3, 4).

DOI: 10.1201/9781032631028-9

Classification

The World Health Organization (WHO) classifies endometrial carcinomas into the following histological subgroups, in descending order of incidence: endometrioid, serous, clear cell, mixed cell adenocarcinoma, undifferentiated, and other rare types including mucinous adenocarcinoma and neuroendocrine tumors (3). The more common histologies are discussed here.

- The **endometrioid** subtype accounts for 70–80% of all endometrioid cancers and is hormonally sensitive, often associated with changes in systemic estrogen acting on the endometrial tissue. Classically, women with endometroid cancers will present with dysfunctional or abnormal uterine bleeding. Endometrioid types of endometrial cancer are commonly associated with deficiencies in mismatch repair proteins (MMRd), though the prevalence is also associated with grade. Up to 70% of low (grade 1–2) tumors are MMRd compared to a 21.5% detection rate in grade 3 endometrioid and an 8.9% in nonendometrioid endometrial cancers (5). When it involves a deficiency in one of the mismatch repair proteins, patients should be screened for Lynch syndrome. However, hypermethylation of the MH2 promoter region also results in MMR deficiency but is not tied to Lynch syndrome. In addition, up to 24% of grade 3 endometrioid cancers express abnormal p53 staining and were associated with an unfavorable survival outcome (6).
- **Uterine serous** carcinoma accounts for 10% of all endometrial cancers and, compared to endometroid cancers, are considered highly aggressive and prone to recurrence when matched for stage (3). Unlike endometrioid cancers they are not associated with estrogen exposure; rather they occur most commonly in the setting of endometrial atrophy (7). They are uniformly considered high-grade cancers and over 90% have abnormal p53 staining (6). Up to 30% are HER2-positive either by protein expression or gene amplification (8).
- **Clear cell** carcinoma accounts for less than 6% of all endometrial cancers and is not hormone-related, exhibiting highly aggressive behavior and poor prognosis, particularly if found at more advanced stages (3).
- As the name suggests, **carcinosarcomas** of the uterus contain both carcinomatous and sarcomatous elements but are staged and treated as high-grade epithelial uterine cancers (3). While various theories have been proposed to explain the appearance of these two disparate tumor histologies, they appear to arise from a monoclonal origin, which explains the treatment paradigm used widely (7).

Molecular Classification of Endometrial Cancer

In 2013, the Cancer Genome Atlas (TCGA) Research Network identified four categories of endometrial carcinomas by molecular features: *POLE* (ultra-mutated) (7%), microsatellite instability (MSI)/hypermutated (28%), copy number low/microsatellite stable (39%), and serous-like/copy number high (26%) (9). These subgroups reflect a better understanding of the clinical and pathologic heterogeneity of endometrial cancer. For example, *POLE* ultra-mutated endometrial carcinomas are associated with a more favorable prognosis, while p53 exhibited unfavorable prognosis (3, 10). Although prospectively validated data are not yet available, these factors have been incorporated into the 2023 clinical staging criteria for endometrial cancer, put forth by the International Federation of Gynecologic Oncology (FIGO, Table 9.1) (11). Notably, the new staging also takes into account histology when assigning stage, distinguishing between non-aggressive (i.e., grade 1 and 2 endometrioid) and aggressive (e.g., serous, clear cell, carcinosarcoma) histologies.

Table 9.1 FIGO Staging of Endometrial Cancer

FIGO Stage	Definition
STAGE I	Confined to the uterine corpus (exception: see IA3)
IA • IA1 • IA2 • IA3	Non-aggressive (1) histologic type with up to 50% involvement of the myometrium Tumor confined to an endometrial polyp or to the endometrium Tumor invades to less than 50% of the myometrium with no evidence of lymphovascular space invasion (LVSI) Low-grade endometrioid adenocarcinoma limited to the uterus **and ovary**
IB	Non-aggressive histologic type invades more than 50% of myometrium with evidence of no more than focal LVSI
IC	Aggressive (1) histologic type limited to a polyp or confined to the endometrium
STAGE II	Tumor invades the cervical stroma or has substantial LVSI or is an aggressive histologic type with myometrial invasion
IIA	Non-aggressive histologic type that invades the cervical stroma
IIB	Non-aggressive histologic type with substantial LVSI
IIC	Aggressive histologic type with any myometrial involvement
STAGE III	Local and/or regional spread of tumor of any histologic type
IIIA • IIIA1 • IIIA2	Tumor invades the uterine serosa, adnexa, or both. Can be by direct extension or established metastases Involvement of the ovary or fallopian tube (excludes stage IA3 disease) Involvement of the uterine subserosa or spread through the uterine serosa
IIIB • IIIB1 • IIIB2	Tumor involves the vagina and/or parametria and/or pelvic peritoneum Metastasis or direct spread to the vagina and/or parametria Metastasis to the pelvic peritoneum
IIIC • IIIC1 • IIIC1i • IIIC1ii • IIIC2 • IIIC2i • IIIC2ii	Metastases to the pelvic and/or para-aortic nodes Metastases confined to the pelvic nodes Microscopic metastatic disease Grossly noted (macroscopic) metastatic disease Metastasis to the para-aortic nodes (with or without pelvic nodes involved) Microscopic Macroscopic
STAGE IV • IVA • IVB • IVC	Spread of tumor to other pelvic organs, abdomen, or more distant disease Invasion of the bladder mucosa and/or intestinal/bowel mucosa Abdominal peritoneal metastases Distant metastases (includes to other intra-abdominal nodes above the renal vessels)

Source: From Berek JS, et al. FIGO staging of endometrial cancer. Int J Gynaecol Obstet 162, 383–394 (2023) Under Creative Commons Attribution license

Note: Aggressive histologies: grade 3 endometrioid, clear cell, serous, carcinosarcoma, and more rare tumor types (undifferentiated, mesonephric-like, gastrointestinal-type mucinous); non-aggressive: grade 1 or 2 endometrioid adenocarcinomas

Approach to Diagnosis and Treatment

The recommended treatment for non-metastatic endometrial cancer is surgery for curative intent, which typically consists of removal of the uterus and cervix, exploration of the abdomen, and sampling of the pelvic and para-aortic nodes. An alternative to the latter is sentinel node biopsy.

For those who undergo surgery, a risk-based strategy is then used to identify patients who should undergo further treatment:

- <u>Low risk</u> is defined as a grade 1–2 tumor of endometrioid or mucinous histology that is confined to the endometrium. These patients are typically observed after surgery, though if there is evidence of a p53 abnormality, the stage is upgraded, which would prompt a discussion of further treatment (e.g., stage IA disease may be upgraded to stage IIc if p53 is abnormal).
- <u>Intermediate risk</u> is associated with low risk factors of any of the following: stage II disease, evidence of lymphovascular invasion of the tumor, lower uterine segment involvement, or over 60 years. These patients are often recommended to pursue a course of radiation therapy. As noted earlier, molecular factors are often used to assign stage of disease. In addition to p53, findings of a hypermutated tumor based on POLE mutation (POLEm) result in downstaging (e.g., stage II disease may be reclassified as stage IA based on POLEm).
- <u>High risk</u> is associated with serous or clear cell cancers of any stage, stage III, or IVa disease of any other histology that has been fully resected. Based on the tumor and patient preferences, it may consist of chemotherapy (carboplatin/paclitaxel in most cases) with or without immunotherapy (dostarlimab or pembrolizumab) (12, 13) with or without the addition of radiation therapy.

For younger patients of child-bearing potential, fertility-sparing options may be available. One example is a person with a grade 1 endometrioid-type endometrial cancer without myometrial infiltration (stage IA). Instead of surgical treatment, hormonal treatment may be attempted in women with early-stage, low-grade disease, particularly as a means of fertility preservation. Additionally, hysteroscopic resection of the tumor and adjacent endometrium can also be done to preserve fertility provided that the disease does not invade the muscle (or myometrium). Otherwise, total hysterectomy with preservation of only the ovaries, if feasible and macroscopically normal, can preserve fertility potential and avoid surgical menopause for younger patients (14).

Cervical Cancer

Epidemiology

Cancer of the uterine cervix is the most frequently diagnosed gynecologic cancer and fourth leading cause of all cancer death in women, with 604,127 new cases and 341,831 deaths worldwide in 2020 (1). Cervical cancer disproportionately affects women in low- and middle-income countries, where access to HPV vaccination, routine pap smears for cervical cancer screening, and treatment services are limited or nonexistent (15). Areas with greatest morbidity and mortality burden of cervical cancer include sub-Saharan Africa, Melanesia, South America, and South-Eastern Asia with 85% of deaths occurring in developing regions of world (16). In the US, 13,820 new cases, and 4,360 deaths are estimated in 2024 (17). Fortunately, the incidence of cervical cancer has decreased by more than half since the mid-1970s due to the widespread uptake of screening and treatment of precursor lesions, but rates have stabilized in recent years (17).

Classification and Staging

Squamous cell carcinoma is the predominant histological subtype of cervical cancer, accounting for 95% of cases, while adenocarcinoma contributes to approximately 5% of invasive cancers worldwide (18). Rarer histologies include clear cell and small cell (or neuroendocrine) tumors. The staging of cervical cancer (19) is provided in Table 9.2.

Table 9.2 FIGO Staging of Cervical Cancer, 2018

STAGE	Definition
STAGE I	Tumor confined to the cervix
IA • IA1 • IA2	Tumor detected only by microscopy; depth of invasion <5 mm Stromal invasion up to 3 mm Stromal invasion >3 and up to 5 mm
IB • IB1 • IB2 • IB3	Tumor invades over 5 mm Tumor size up to 2 cm Tumor size >2 and up to 4 cm Tumor measures over 4 cm
STAGE II	Tumor invades beyond the uterus but does not extend distally to the lower vagina nor does it involve the pelvic sidewall
IIA • IIA1 • IIA2	Involvement is limited to upper two thirds of the vagina, no parametrial invasion Tumor size up to 4 cm Tumor >4 cm
IIB	Parametrial invasion noted but not to the side wall
STAGE III	Tumor extends into the lower vagina, impacts the ureters, or involves nodes
IIIA	Extension limited to the lower third of the vagina
IIIB	Extension to the pelvic wall and/or is associated with hydronephrosis or a non-functioning kidney
IIIC • IIIC1 • IIIC2	Extension to the lymph nodes Pelvic node metastases only Para-aortic node metastases
STAGE IV	Extends beyond the true pelvis
IVA	Involves adjacent pelvic organs
IVB	Spread to distant organs

Source: (From Bhatla N, Aoki D, Sharma DN et al. Cancer of the cervix uteri: 2021 update. Int J Gynaecol Obstet 155 Suppl 1, 28–44 (2021) with permission)

Approach to Diagnosis and Treatment

The diagnosis of cervical cancer is made by histologic confirmation of invasion. If there is no visible lesion, it is often made following colposcopy. For all people diagnosed with cervical cancer, a PET/CT is often performed to assess the extent of disease, including to the pelvic and para-aortic nodes, and more distally to the supraclavicular node. The treatment for invasive disease is outlined based on the extent of disease. When PET/CT is not available, standard procedures in the staging of cervical cancer include a contrast CT of the chest, abdomen, and pelvis, hysteroscopy, endoscopy, and proctoscopy. In cases in which kidney involvement is suspected, an intravenous pyelogram (IVP) can be used in lieu of CT.

For women with limited disease (i.e., stage IA up to IB2) of more common histologies (e.g., squamous or adenocarcinoma), the options can include conization or radical trachelectomy as a means to preserve the uterus for future fertility. For those who present with more advanced disease, fertility-sparing approaches are not an option.

For those who have early-stage disease (up to IB2), the treatment is surgical consisting of a radical hysterectomy and node dissection (or sampling). Postoperatively, adjuvant radiation is indicated based on a combination of specific pathologic features commonly referred to as the Sedlis criteria, namely the depth of stromal invasion, presence of lymphovascular space invasion, and tumor size (20). For others whose tumors are associated with pathologic involvement of the lymph nodes, parametrial involvement, or when tumor is present at the surgical margins (the Peters criteria), chemotherapy with radiation is indicated (21).

People found to have a cervical lesion that measures 4 cm or larger (stage IB3) are referred to as having a "barrel-shaped lesion." These patients no longer are taken to the operating room and instead are treated with chemoradiation with curative intent (definitive therapy) using the chemotherapy agent cisplatin on a weekly basis to sensitize the tumor to radiotherapy (22). For those whose tumors extend locally (to the lower vaginal wall, pelvic sidewall, or are associated with hydronephrosis, FIGO Stage III) the US Food and Drug Administration has granted the approval for the use of pembrolizumab, an immune checkpoint inhibitor (23). Importantly, this approval is limited to those patients *without* lymph node involvement. In the presence of lymph node involvement, pembrolizumab is not indicated; chemoradiation is the standard recommendation with radiation fields designed to cover the nodes involved and at risk (often in the para-aortic chain).

Younger patients who have ovarian function and who are recommended for pelvic radiation are candidates for ovarian transposition (oophoropexy) with the aim to retain ovarian function by suspending the gonads above the iliac crests and out of the radiation field. While data are limited it does appear to be effective. In a 2023 systematic review of ovarian transposition prior to pelvic RT for younger women with an anorectal malignancy, the pooled proportion that had intact ovarian function was 66.9% (95% CI, 55–79%) (24). This is with an older systematic review that focused specifically on people treated for gynecologic cancers in whom the rate of incidence of preserved ovarian function following external beam RT was 65% (95% CI 56–74%) (25).

Ovarian Cancer

Epidemiology

Ovarian cancer is the third most common gynecologic cancer diagnosed in women globally, with 313,959 new cases and 207,252 deaths in 2020 (1). Incidence rates are highest among non-Hispanic White women, 30% higher than non-Hispanic Blacks (NHB) and Asian American/Pacific Islanders (AAPI) (26). Despite being less frequent than endometrial and cervical cancers, it remains the most fatal of the gynecologic cancers due to its high propensity for detection only when disease has left the ovary. Fortunately, strides have been made in the classification and the approach of ovarian cancer with an accompanying improvement in survival outcomes.

Classification and Staging

Cancers arising in the ovary can be epithelial and non-epithelial in origin. The most common is high-grade serous epithelial ovarian cancer, which is typically diagnosed in women older than 70 (27). In contrast, low-grade serous carcinoma (LGSC) presents in women in their 50s most often and constitutes up to 5% of all epithelial ovarian cancers. Compared to HGSC they carry a better prognosis (ten-year survival of 70% vs. 26%) (27). Other types of epithelial ovarian cancers include endometrioid (10%), mucinous (6%), and clear cell (6%), with the remaining 25% being more rare subtypes or unspecified (26).

Non-epithelial cancers are less common and less aggressive than epithelial cancers of the ovary. These include germ cell and sex cord-stromal tumor, accounting for 3% and 2% of all ovarian

Table 9.3 FIGO Staging of Ovarian Cancer, 2018

STAGE	*DEFINITION*
STAGE I	Tumor limited to the ovaries
IA	Tumor limited to one ovary with capsule intact or in the fallopian tube without surface involvement; no malignant cells in ascites
IB	Tumor involves both ovaries with capsules intact or fallopian tubes with no surface involvement; no malignant cells in ascites
IC • IC1 • IC2 • IC3	Tumor involving one or both ovaries Surgical spill Capsule rupture Malignant ascites
STAGE II	Tumor with pelvic extension
IIA	Extension and/or implants to the uterus, tubes, and/or ovaries
IIB	Extension to other tissues in the true pelvis
STAGE III	Tumor extends to the abdomen +/- retroperitoneal node involvement

IIIA
• IIIA
  • IIIAi
  • IIIAii
	Microscopic peritoneal involvement
	Positive retroperitoneal nodes
	Nodal metastasis up to 10 mm in greatest dimension
	Nodal metastasis >10 mm in greatest dimension

IIIB	Macroscopic peritoneal involvement 2 cm or less
IIIC	Macroscopic peritoneal involvement >2 cm
STAGE IV	Distant metastases
IVA	Pleural cytology positive for malignancy
IVB	Other organ involvement (including inguinal nodes and nodes outside the abdominal cavity)

Source: (Adapted from Amin MB, Edge SB, Greene FL, et al., eds, AJCC [American Joint Committee on Cancer] Cancer Staging Manual, Springer, Chicago, IL, 2018)

cancers, respectively. Generally, non-epithelial types have a younger age distribution, and most are diagnosed early, which carries an excellent prognosis (26). Staging typically consists of a CT scan of the chest, abdomen, and pelvis, but the diagnosis is often made at the time of surgery. The staging system of ovarian cancer is given in Table 9.3 (28).

Approach to Diagnosis and Treatment

The primary treatment of ovarian cancer is surgical, and the goal of surgery is the removal of all disease, called an optimal cytoreduction. For those in whom an optimal surgical result is doubtful at the time of presentation, or for people in whom the risks of surgery are significant, neoadjuvant chemotherapy consisting of a platinum-based combination is often recommended. This approach is associated with less perioperative morbidity without risking inferior survival outcomes (29).

Chemotherapy for ovarian cancer typically consists of a platinum-taxane-based combination (e.g., carboplatin and paclitaxel), particularly for epithelial ovarian cancers. Although most patients will receive treatment, those with very early disease confined to the ovary (stage IA) may elect for surveillance only given the excellent prognosis with definitive surgery.

For people with non-epithelial ovarian cancer, medical treatment is typically guided by specific factors based on histologic type, such as stage IC or higher granulosa cell tumors, poorly differentiated or higher stage Sertoli-Leydig tumors, and most diagnosed with ovarian germ-cell tumors regardless of stage. Cisplatin and etoposide (EP) with or without bleomycin (BEP) is often the regimen of choice for these patients. One randomized trial enrolled people with newly diagnosed (stage II to IV) or recurrent sex cord-stromal tumors and compared BEP to carboplatin and paclitaxel. Although closed due to futility, it suggested that carboplatin/paclitaxel was as effective and less toxic (30).

Genetic Testing

One of the biggest advances in epithelial ovarian cancer was the recognition of genetic mutations that confer risk of developing this disease, in addition to breast cancer. BRCA1 and BRCA2 are the most common genetic mutations and contribute to approximately 18% of epithelial ovarian cancers, especially high-grade serous subtype (31). BRCA1 and BRCA 2 mutations confer a 44% and 17% increased risk of developing ovarian cancer by the age of 80, respectively (32). The added importance of identifying people with ovarian cancer associated with BRCA1/2 mutations is that they are eligible for additional treatment (or maintenance) following completion of chemotherapy with a Poly-ADP-Ribose-Polymerase (PARP) inhibitor. Two studies showed that the use of PARP inhibitors in this setting is associated with significantly improved progression-free survival (33).

Gestational Trophoblast Neoplasia

Epidemiology

While rare, gestational trophoblastic diseases (GTDs) are almost exclusively diagnosed in women of reproductive age, and they occur with a bimodal distribution affecting women under 20 or over 40, and particularly in those over the age of 45 (34). The incidence of hydatidiform moles vary globally, with rates of 1–2 per 1,000 pregnancies in Europe and North America compared to 10 per 1,000 in regions such as India and Indonesia. Factors such as genetics and diet may contribute to these differences, with higher reported frequencies of GTDs in areas with greater risk for malnutrition (35, 36). The likelihood of developing an invasive mole rises significantly, up to 40–50%, in patients with specific risk factors: age greater than 40, uterine size exceeding the expected gestational age by more than four weeks, human chorionic gonadotropin (hCG) levels of 100,000 mIU/mL or higher, and the presence of bilateral theca lutein cysts measuring 6 cm or greater (37). Choriocarcinomas occur at a rate of about 1 per 40,000 pregnancies in Europe and North America, while in Southeast Asia, the incidence is higher, at 9.2 per 40,000 pregnancies. Approximately 25% of choriocarcinoma cases follow pregnancy loss or ectopic pregnancy, another 25% are associated with term or preterm gestations, and the remaining 50% arise from hydatidiform moles. However, only 2% to 3% of hydatidiform moles are estimated to progress to choriocarcinoma (35). Although estimates vary, choriocarcinomas are most commonly associated with complete hydatidiform moles (CHM), are rare after partial hydatidiform moles (PHM), and may occur in 2 to 7 per 100,000 other pregnancies. Placental site trophoblastic tumor (PSTT) accounts for approximately 0.2% of all GTD cases, while ETTs remain even more seldom in occurrence (38, 39).

Classification and Staging

Gestational trophoblastic disease (GTD) encompasses a group of related conditions that are generally classified into two categories: gestational trophoblastic disease (GTD) and gestational trophoblastic neoplasia (GTN), the latter being the primary focus of this section. GTDs represent abnormal proliferations of placental tissue, including exaggerated placental site reactions, placental site nodules, and hydatidiform moles. In contrast, GTNs are tumors arising from extravillous trophoblasts with varying degrees of malignancy, such as invasive moles, choriocarcinomas, placental site trophoblastic tumors (PSTT), and epithelioid trophoblastic tumors (ETT).

An invasive mole, often considered a malignant form of GTD, is typically diagnosed clinically rather than pathologically, based on the persistent elevation of human chorionic gonadotropin (hCG) following molar evacuation (40). Choriocarcinomas are a malignant condition marked by abnormal trophoblastic hyperplasia and anaplasia, the absence of chorionic villi, and the presence of hemorrhage and necrosis, with direct invasion into the myometrium and vascular structures. Placental site trophoblastic tumors (PSTT) involve malignant proliferation of intermediate trophoblasts at the site of placental implantation. Finally, the epithelioid trophoblastic tumor (ETT) is the rarest form of gestational trophoblastic tumor, arising from the malignant transformation of intermediate trophoblasts at the chorionic level (41). GTD is subsequently staged according to FIGO criteria, aided by the World Health Organization (WHO) prognostic scoring system (Table 9.4) (42).

Approach to Diagnosis and Treatment

The diagnosis of a GTN following a molar pregnancy is based on elevated human chorionic gonadotropin (hCG) levels, and both imaging and pathology can support the diagnosis. Unlike

Table 9.4   FIGO Staging of Gestational Trophoblast Neoplasia and the Modified WHO Prognostic Scoring System

STAGE	DEFINITION			
STAGE I	Disease confined to the uterus			
STAGE II	Disease extends to the genital structures only (e.g., adnexa, vagina)			
STAGE III	Disease involves the lungs			
STAGE IV	All other metastatic sites			
WHO RISK FACTOR	SCORE			
	0	1	2	4
Age (years)	<40	≥40	—	—
Antecedent pregnancy	Mole	Abortion	Term	—
Interval to diagnosis (months)	<4	4–6	7–12	>12
Pretreatment serum hCG (mIU/mL)	$<10^3$	10^3 to 10^4	10^4 to 10^5	$>10^5$
Largest tumor size (cm)	<3	3–4	≥5	—
Site of metastases	Lung	Spleen, Kidney	GI tract	Brain, Liver
Number of metastases	—	1 to 4	5 to 8	≥8
Prior lines of treatment	—	—	Single drug	≥2

Source: (From Berkowitz RS, Goldstein DP. Current management of gestational trophoblastic diseases. Gynecol Oncol 112, 654–662 (2009) with permission)

other solid tumors, a tissue biopsy is not required before initiating treatment. The interpretation of hCG levels varies depending on the patient's history of molar pregnancy. After the evacuation of a complete or partial molar pregnancy, hCG levels are monitored weekly until they become undetectable. If hCG levels either rise or remain stable over several weeks, post molar GTN is diagnosed using criteria from the International Federation of Gynecology and Obstetrics (FIGO). These criteria include hCG levels plateauing over a three-week period, or increasing by more than 10% across three measurements taken over two weeks (43). Subsequently, the diagnosis of a GTN following a nonmolar pregnancy is made based on elevated hCG levels, once other possible causes such as a normal viable pregnancy, abnormal pregnancies, ectopic hCG production by a non-trophoblastic tumor, or other causes of low-level hCG production have been ruled out (44). Evidence of likely metastatic disease supports the diagnosis, and extrauterine biopsies are not recommended due to risk of promoting life-threatening hemorrhage upon biopsy (45, 46).

A WHO score of 0 to 6 is indicative of low-risk disease, and treatment is often with single-agent methotrexate or actinomycin D. Scores above 6 indicate higher-risk disease and combination chemotherapy is often utilized. Given the complexity in management of GTD, referral to a specialized center is strongly suggested.

Survivorship Issues after Gynecologic Cancer Treatment

There are over 1.4 million gynecologic cancer survivors in the US, and this number is only expected to increase (47–49). The prevalence of gynecologic cancers is increasing due to an aging population, increased rates of risk factors such as obesity (50), and increasing survival rates (51). Gynecologic survivors experience high rates of a second cancer (52) due to shared risk factors such as obesity, tobacco, and genetics, so engaging survivors in healthy lifestyle and weight changes and cancer screening is essential. Gynecologic cancer survivors report a number of issues post treatment including issues with fatigue, sleep, sexual concerns, neurologic symptoms, bladder and bowel dysfunction, and higher rates of depression and anxiety (49, 51) all of which not only impact quality of life, but can create barriers to healthy lifestyle changes. While not specific to women experiencing menopausal symptoms following gynecologic cancer treatment, they are universal issues that require commentary in any discussion on survivorship.

Healthy Lifestyles

All cancer survivors should engage in regular moderate physical activity (minimum of 150 minutes of moderate activity/week) (53), eat a diet rich in whole grains, fruits and vegetables, and legumes, and low intake of meat and processed foods (54), and maintain or achieve normal body mass index (BMI). Lifestyle interventions for weight loss among gynecologic cancer survivors have had mixed results (55), although some studies have shown modest success (56, 57). Observational data suggest that GLP-1 agonists may reduce the incidence of obesity-related cancers (58), but their use is still recommended only for cancer survivors with a diagnosis of diabetes or those who have not had success at weight control with other interventions (59). Gynecologic cancer survivors who exercise regularly do appear to have reduced fatigue, anxiety and depression, and improved quality of life (QoL) (57, 60, 61). A structured cardiac rehabilitation program among cancer survivors at high risk of cardiovascular outcomes has been shown to improve cardiac function, cardiovascular risk factor control, and QoL (62).

A systematic review of interventions to improve healthy eating among cancer patients has shown improvement in self-reported fruit and vegetable intake and adiposity (63). While interventions varied in length and content, they employed the use of education materials, classes or counseling sessions, diet-relevant supplies, and logbooks or website tools to track food consumption. However, more research is needed to identify specific aspects of interventions that are most effective in promoting change.

Fatigue

Cancer-related fatigue is a common complaint among cancer survivors that has been defined as "a persistent, often overwhelming feeling of physical, mental, and/or emotional exhaustion" (64). Estimates of prevalence of fatigue among gynecologic cancer survivors range from 44.3% (65) to 54% (66) and are highest within the first six months of treatment completion. Fatigue remains high among a significant proportion of patients years after treatment (67).

Assessment of fatigue includes identifying and treating contributing factors such as poor sleep quality due to pain, vasomotor symptoms, and obstructive sleep apnea, as well as depression and anxiety. Interventions to improve fatigue include physical exercise (68), cognitive behavioral therapy (CBT), yoga (69), and education interventions (70). Stimulants and wakefulness agents are not recommended for fatigue in cancer survivors (68).

Sexual Dysfunction

Sexual dysfunction is increased among gynecologic survivors (71, 72). Surgery, radiation, and chemotherapy, as well as changes in body image all can impact sexual function and desire. The rates of sexual dysfunction (including dyspareunia, vaginal dryness, and vaginitis) among gynecologic cancers has been reported to be 2.5 times higher than that of age-matched controls (73). Decreased sexual satisfaction among gynecologic cancer survivors (65%) is common, with arousal and pain with penetration being the most frequently reported complaints (71).

Concerns related to pain with penetrative sexual activities (dyspareunia) should prompt a complete pelvic exam with attention to any evidence of recurrence, vaginal stenosis, prolapse of pelvic floor organs, pelvic floor dysfunction, vaginal atrophy, and dryness.

Decreased libido is challenging to address but attention to mitigating or eliminating other issues, such as dyspareunia, is essential. Diagnosing and treating vaginismus as well as vaginal dryness can help improve sexual desire. Vaginal dryness can be treated with topical estrogen which is generally considered safe after gynecologic cancer. Alternative hormonal preparations including topical prasterone, and the consistent use of vaginal moisturizers are also key. These interventions should be complemented by the liberal use of lubricants during sexual activity. Pain that is limited to the vestibule can be effectively treated with 4% aqueous lidocaine. This was shown in a small randomized trial in women previously treated for breast cancer (74) but can apply to those treated for gynecologic cancers as well.

Treatments for provoked pelvic floor hypertonus (vaginismus) include pelvic floor physical therapy and the use of dilators. A patient's partner should be part of the treatment plan to address sexual concerns and if relationship conflict is present, then couple's counseling can be helpful as well. Flibanserin is an FDA-approved medication to treat hypoactive sexual desire disorder, but side effects of low blood pressure, fatigue and dizziness, and the need to abstain from alcohol, as well as the lack of data in cancer survivors, have limited its use.

Vasomotor Symptoms

For those who are premenopausal or perimenopausal at the time of diagnosis, removal of the ovaries, pelvic radiation, and some chemotherapy agents can thrust them into premature ovarian failure. Indeed, some data indicate that surgically induced menopause causes more intensive and intrusive symptoms than natural menopause (75).

In general, people treated for gynecologic cancer are candidates for hormone therapy (HT). In a 2016 meta-analysis that included six randomized trials conducted in people with a history of ovarian cancer (n = 1,521), compared to those who did not receive HT, its use was associated with a significantly lower risk of ovarian cancer-related death (OR 0.47, 95% CI 0.28–0.80) and had no impact on recurrence rates (OR 0.71, 95% CI 0.45–1.14) or on overall survival outcomes (76). Importantly, these data do not readily apply to hormonally mediated tumors, such as ovarian low-grade serous carcinoma and granulosa cell tumors, and low-grade endometrial stromal sarcoma of the uterus. Barakat et al. conducted GOG 137, which enrolled volunteers with stage I/II endometrial cancer (n = 1,236) and randomly assigned them to estrogen therapy or placebo. The study was stopped early, but at three years, there was no difference in overall or progression-free survival, nor was there a significant risk of recurrence with estrogen compared to placebo (RR 1.27, 80% CI 0.92–1.77) (77). Finally, a randomized trial in cervical cancer was conducted in the late 1980s and evaluated HT (dienestrol and chlormadinone) versus no HT. There was no statistically significant difference in either the five-year survival or recurrence rates (78). These data were subsequently confirmed in a 2021 meta-analysis (79). Unfortunately, single institutional data suggest that fewer than half of women who are eligible for HT are counseled or prescribed HT (80).

For those who are either not good candidates for hormone replacement therapy after diagnosis, non-hormonal options include serotonin reuptake inhibitors (SSRIs), serotonin norepinephrine reuptake inhibitors (SNRIs), gabapentin, and clonidine. There is currently one neurokinin 3 (NK3) receptor antagonist approved by the FDA and another in development which are non-hormonal options as well. Cognitive behavioral therapy (CBT) and stellate ganglion blocks have shown promise in reducing symptoms (71, 81). Acupuncture has had mixed or conflicting results (82) but is safe and well tolerated, and limited data suggest that hypnotherapy may also palliate (83).

Urinary Symptoms

Urinary symptoms are reported commonly among gynecologic cancer survivors (50, 84, 85). Surgery, radiation, hormonal changes, and chemotherapy may all potentially cause or contribute to urinary symptoms. Stress urinary incontinence rates range from 24% to 36% and urge incontinence rates from 8% to 25% (85). A pelvic exam to help identify prolapse or vaginal atrophy and a urinalysis to identify infections should be performed to identify contributing urinary symptoms. Lifestyle changes and bladder training, pelvic floor physical therapy, and medications can all be helpful in managing incontinence symptoms (50). Interstitial cystitis can appear years after cancer treatment is completed and causes significant pain and disability. Physical therapy for those with pelvic floor tenderness, amitriptyline, and pentosan polysulfate are options for pharmacologic treatment.

Neuropathy

Chemotherapy-induced peripheral neuropathy (CIPN) is a common side effect of treatment with taxane and platinum-based chemotherapy regimens (86) and can persist for years after treatment

(84). Evaluation of CIPN should include evaluating for any contributing factors (B vitamin deficiencies, thyroid disorders, or metabolic disorders). Duloxetine has the best evidence for alleviating the symptoms of CIPN (87) but exercise (88) and acupuncture (50) show promise as well. Supportive footwear and physical therapy may also be helpful (50). SSRIs and SNRIs may ameliorate concomitant depression due to chronic pain as an added benefit.

Psychosocial Concerns

Similar to people treated for other cancers, survivors from a gynecologic malignancy experience anxiety, depression, fear of recurrence, and uncertainty about the future (84). Prevalence of depression estimates range from 23% to 27% and anxiety 19–33% (65, 89, 90). Treatment for depression and anxiety in cancer survivors is based on severity of symptoms and impairment. Supportive care can and should be offered to all cancer survivors with depression and anxiety. Those with moderate symptoms can be referred to group or individual therapy which can include CBT, mindfulness and stress-reduction, behavioral activation, exercise programs, and medication if patients fail to improve. Patients with severe depression should be offered individual therapy and medication if they do not have access to therapy, prefer pharmacotherapy, or fail to respond to non-pharmacologic interventions. First-line medications to treat depression include SSRI and SNRIs, although a recent panel from the American Society of Clinical Oncology concluded that there are little data to inform the benefits of medications for cancer-related psychologic distress (91).

Table 9.5   Common Survivorship Issues Experienced by Gynecologic Cancer Survivors, Provider Assessment, Resources, and Tools

Survivorship Issue	Provider Screening Resources/Tools	Assessment/Recommendations
Surveillance for secondary cancers	NCCN site-specific survivorship guidelines ACS USPSTF	History and physical exam Age-based screening for all cancers modified by: Genetic/familial high risk-based screening recs (e.g., BRCA, FAP) Treatment exposure (pelvic radiation and risk for skin and sarcomas, and colorectal cancer (pelvic XRT < age 30) Shared exposures (HPV, tobacco)
Healthy lifestyle	NCCN survivorship screening questions for diet and exercise "Tell me about your diet." "What have you eaten in the last 24 hours? Is this typical?" "In the past month, was there any day when you or anyone in your family went hungry because you did not have enough money for food?"	Screen for barriers to healthy lifestyle Fatigue, anemia, neuropathy, food insecurity 150 to 300 minutes moderate-intensity exercise weekly Diet rich in whole grains and fruits, low in saturated fats and processed foods Nutritionist referral State and medical center-specific programming

(Continued)

Table 9.5 *(Continued)* **Common Survivorship Issues Experienced by Gynecologic Cancer Survivors, Provider Assessment, Resources, and Tools**

Survivorship Issue	Provider Screening Resources/Tools	Assessment/Recommendations
Fatigue	NCCN survivorship questions PROMIS 8-item scale for fatigue	Screen: depression, anemia, pain, vitamin deficiency, electrolyte abnormalities, metabolic disorders, poor sleep habits, OSA, cardiac or pulmonary disease, autoimmune disorders as indicated Treatment: CBT Encourage graded physical activity Conservation of energy Cancer rehabilitation provider (PT or MD)
Sexual dysfunction	NCCN survivorship questions PROMIS Brief Profile for Sexual Function and Satisfaction FSFI-6	Screen: gynecological exam for atrophic changes, vaginismus, vaginal infections, and cancer recurrence Depression and anxiety Evaluate relationship status, contributing medications (SSRIs, SNRIs) Treatment: Vaginal moisturizers (including topical estrogen), lubricants Pelvic floor PT, trained sex therapist (by AASECT https://www.aasect.org/) Bupropion, flibanserin (premenopausal)
Vasomotor symptoms	NCCN survivorship questions	Assess and treat: frequency, intensity, and impact on sleep or other activities Treatment: SSRIs, SNRIs, gabapentin, fezolinetant Acupuncture
Urinary symptoms	NCCN survivorship questions Categorize stress, urge, or mixed incontinence	Screen: gynecologic exam, vaginal cultures, urinalysis, contributing medications (diuretics, antidepressants, alpha blockers) Treatment: Lifestyle changes Bladder training, antimuscarinics, mirabegron, botulinum injection, Pelvic floor physical therapy
Neuropathy	NCCN survivorship questions	Screen: nutritional deficiencies (B12, folate) metabolic (A1c, TSH, autoimmune if indicated) Treatment: Physical therapy (balance training) Duloxetine, gabapentin, pregabalin, tricyclics Acupuncture

(Continued)

Table 9.5 *(Continued)* **Common Survivorship Issues Experienced by Gynecologic Cancer Survivors, Provider Assessment, Resources, and Tools**

Survivorship Issue	Provider Screening Resources/Tools	Assessment/Recommendations
Psychosocial issues	PHQ-9, GAD-7, PHQ-4 (combined depression and anxiety screen) Distress thermometer HITS screener for IPV	Screen: depression and anxiety, intimate partner violence, and substance use, financial toxicity Treatment: CBT, support groups Medications (SSRIs, SNRIs)
Sleep	PROMIS sleep 4a	Screen: pain, anxiety, sleep disorders, hot flashes, substance use Treatment: CBT and sleep hygiene Short-term use of sleep medications (ramelteon, dual orexin receptor antagonists, doxepin)
Financial toxicity	COST 12-item scale "Have you had financial (money) problems due to your cancer or costs related to your cancer?"	Referral to social work or other hospital or community-based resources
Fertility concerns	NCCN survivorship questions	Appropriate assessment and referral based on treatments received If early stage and reproductive organs intact cannot assume infertile Referral to fertility specialist (can search via ASRM website)

Note: (Chapter Appendix lists resources for patients)

Fear of recurrence and cancer-specific worry are common (39–97%) among cancer survivors with nearly half reporting moderate to severe worry (92, 93). Among a cohort of gynecologic cancer survivors, 30% scored high in cancer recurrence worry (94). While fear of recurrence decreases over time for most, it remains elevated in a significant proportion of long-term survivors (95). Interventions such as CBT that focus on processes of cognition (worry rumination and attentional bias) can be particularly effective (96). Mindfulness-based exercises and creative therapies like art and writing may be helpful for managing these symptoms as well (50).

Conclusions

Menopausal symptoms that arise in people treated for gynecologic cancers should be viewed in context of their disease characteristics and treatments, since the differential risk to the ovaries with surgery, chemotherapy, and/or radiation vary by disease origin. These symptoms should also be viewed in the context of the larger survivorship issues as we help people adjust to life after cancer and attain their new normal. In general, HT is not contraindicated following treatment of gynecologic cancers, although caveats exist. Sadly, these statements are not driven by high-quality evidence, but rather the consensus of experts in the field. Further work is required to better delineate the risks and benefits of HT after treatments for these tumors.

Appendix: Patient Resources

General Guidelines for Late and Long-Term Effects for Cancer Survivors

* NCCN: https://www.nccn.org/patients/guidelines/content/PDF/survivorship-crl-patient.pdf
* NCI "Facing Forward": https://www.cancer.gov/publications/patient-education/life-after-treatment.pdf

Physical Activity and Nutrition

■ YMCA "Live-Strong" programs (available at some YMCAs)
■ MyPlate: https://www.myplate.gov/
■ ACS: https://www.cancer.org/content/dam/cancer-org/cancer-control/en/booklets-flyers/nutrition-and-physical-activity-after-cancer-treatment.pdf
■ ACS app: ACS Cares available at APP store
■ NCCN: www.nccn.org/patients/guidelines/content/PDF/survivorship-hl-patient.pdf

Cancer-Specific Organizations

■ Society of Gynecologic Oncology, Survivorship Toolkit: https://www.sgo.org/survivorship-toolkit/
■ National Ovarian Cancer Coalition: Online Education Programs: https://ovarian.org/programs-and-resources/nocc-online-education-programs/

Survivorship Clinics

■ NCI designated cancer centers: https://www.cancer.gov/research/infrastructure/cancer-centers

Community Access to Resources, Education, and Support

■ ACS patient programs and other programs and services: https://www.cancer.org/support-programs-and-services.html
■ Phone app "ACS Cares"

Local Hospital and Cancer Centers
Peer Support

■ Cancer Survivors Network (ovarian, endometrial, and other gynecologic cancer specific chat/support): https://csn.cancer.org/

Fertility

■ ASRM: Patient information: www.reproductivefacts.org/

Guidelines for Cancer Survivorship (Providers)

* NCCN: www.nccn.org/professionals/physician_gls/pdf/survivorship.pdf

References

1. Sung H et al. Global cancer statistics 2020: GLOBOCAN estimates of incidence and mortality worldwide for 36 cancers in 185 countries. CA Cancer J Clin. 2021;71:209–49.
2. Koskas M et al. Cancer of the corpus uteri: 2021 update. Int J Gynecol Obstet (Wiley Online Library). 2021 Oct;155(1_suppl):45–60.
3. Yen TT et al. Molecular classification and emerging targeted therapy in endometrial cancer. Int J Gynecol Pathol. 2020;39:26–35.
4. Garg K, Soslow RA. Endometrial carcinoma in women aged 40 years and younger. Arch Pathol Lab Med. 2014;138:335–42.
5. Loukovaara M et al. Mismatch repair deficiency as a predictive and prognostic biomarker in molecularly classified endometrial carcinoma. Cancers. 2021;13:3124.
6. Jamieson A et al. p53abn Endometrial cancer: Understanding the most aggressive endometrial cancers in the era of molecular classification. Int J Gynecol Cancer. 2021;31:907–13.
7. Bell DW, Ellenson LH. Molecular genetics of endometrial carcinoma. Annu Rev Pathol. 2019;14:339–67.
8. Buza N. HER2 testing in endometrial serous carcinoma: Time for standardized pathology practice to meet the clinical demand. Arch Pathol Lab Med. 2021;145:687–91.
9. Network CG et al. Integrated genomic characterization of endometrial carcinoma. Nature. 2013;497:67–73.
10. Stelloo E et al. Practical guidance for mismatch repair-deficiency testing in endometrial cancer. Ann Oncol. 2017;28:96–102.
11. Berek JS et al. FIGO staging of endometrial cancer: 2023. Int J Gynaecol Obstet. 2023;162:383–94.
12. Mirza MR et al. Dostarlimab for primary advanced or recurrent endometrial cancer. N Engl J Med. 2023;388:2145–58.
13. Eskander RN et al. Pembrolizumab plus chemotherapy in advanced endometrial cancer. N Engl J Med. 2023;388:2159–70.
14. Pessini SA et al. Fertility preservation in gynecologic cancer patients. Rev Bras Ginecol Obstet. 2023;45:161–8.
15. WHO/ICO Information Center of HPV and Cervical Cancer (HPV Information Center). Human papillomavirus and related cancers in the world. Summary Report. 2010.
16. Pimple S, Mishra G. Cancer cervix: Epidemiology and disease burden. J Cytol. 2022;19.
17. Siegel RL et al. Cancer statistics, 2024. CA Cancer J Clin. 2024;74:12–49.
18. Fowler M et al. Cervical cancer. In: StatPearls. StatPearls Publishing; 2024.
19. Bhatla N et al. Cancer of the cervix uteri: 2021 update. Int J Gynaecol Obstet. 2021;155(1_suppl):28–44.
20. Sedlis A et al. A randomized trial of pelvic radiation therapy versus no further therapy in selected patients with stage IB carcinoma of the cervix after radical hysterectomy and pelvic lymphadenectomy: A gynecologic oncology group study. Gynecol Oncol. 1999;73:177–83.
21. Peters WA et al. Concurrent chemotherapy and pelvic radiation therapy compared with pelvic radiation therapy alone as adjuvant therapy after radical surgery in high-risk early-stage cancer of the cervix. J Clin Oncol. 2000;18:1606–13.
22. Chemoradiotherapy for Cervical Cancer Meta-analysis Collaboration (CCCMAC). Reducing uncertainties about the effects of chemoradiotherapy for cervical cancer: Individual patient data meta-analysis. Cochrane Database Syst Rev. 2010;CD008285. doi:10.1002/14651858.CD008285.
23. Lorusso D et al. Pembrolizumab or placebo with chemoradiotherapy followed by pembrolizumab or placebo for newly diagnosed, high-risk, locally advanced cervical cancer (ENGOT-cx11/GOG-3047/KEYNOTE-A18): A randomised, double-blind, phase 3 clinical trial. Lancet. 2024;403:1341–50.
24. Tessier L et al. Laparoscopic ovarian transposition prior to pelvic radiation in young women with anorectal malignancies: A systematic review and meta-analysis of prevalence. Colorectal Dis. 2023;25:1336–48.
25. Gubbala K et al. Outcomes of ovarian transposition in gynaecological cancers: A systematic review and meta-analysis. J Ovarian Res. 2014;7:69.
26. Torre LA et al. Ovarian cancer statistics, 2018. CA Cancer J Clin. 2018;68:284–96.

27. Babaier A et al. Low-grade serous carcinoma of the ovary: The current status. Diagnostics (Basel). 2022;12:458.
28. Amin MB et al., eds. AJCC (American Joint Committee on Cancer) Cancer Staging Manual. Chicago, IL: Springer; 2018.
29. Wright AA et al. Use and effectiveness of intraperitoneal chemotherapy for treatment of ovarian cancer. J Clin Oncol. 2015. doi:10.1200/JCO.2015.61.4776.
30. Schultz KAP et al. Ovarian sex cord-stromal tumors. J Oncol Pract. 2016;12:940–6.
31. Norquist BM et al. Inherited mutations in women with ovarian carcinoma. JAMA Oncol. 2016;2:482–90.
32. Kuchenbaecker KB et al. Risks of breast, ovarian, and contralateral breast cancer for BRCA1 and BRCA2 mutation carriers. JAMA. 2017;317:2402–16.
33. Tattersall A et al. Poly(ADP-ribose) polymerase (PARP) inhibitors for the treatment of ovarian cancer. Cochrane Database Syst Rev. 2022;2:CD007929.
34. Melamed A et al. Effect of race/ethnicity on risk of complete and partial molar pregnancy after adjustment for age. Gynecol Oncol. 2016;143:73–6.
35. Eysbouts YK et al. Trends in incidence for gestational trophoblastic disease over the last 20years in a population-based study. Gynecol Oncol. 2016;140:70–5.
36. Strohl AE, Lurain JR. Clinical epidemiology of gestational trophoblastic disease. Curr Obstet Gynecol Rep. 2014;3:40–3.
37. Elias KM et al. Complete hydatidiform mole in women aged 40 to 49 years. J Reprod Med. 2012;57:254–8.
38. Joyce CM et al. Advances in the diagnosis and early management of gestational trophoblastic disease. BMJ Med. 2022;1:e000321.
39. Schmid P et al. Prognostic markers and long-term outcome of placental-site trophoblastic tumours: A retrospective observational study. Lancet. 2009;374:48–55.
40. Seckl MJ et al. Gestational trophoblastic disease. Lancet. 2010;376:717–29.
41. Hui P. Gestational trophoblastic tumors: A timely review of diagnostic pathology. Arch Pathol Lab Med. 2019;143:65–74.
42. Berkowitz RS, Goldstein DP. Current management of gestational trophoblastic diseases. Gynecol Oncol. 2009;112:654–62.
43. Ngan HY et al. Gestational trophoblastic neoplasia, FIGO 2000 staging and classification. Int J Gynaecol Obstet. 2003;83(1_suppl):175–7.
44. Harvey RA et al. Differences in total human chorionic gonadotropin immunoassay analytical specificity and ability to measure human chorionic gonadotropin in gestational trophoblastic disease and germ cell tumors. J Reprod Med. 2010;55:285–95.
45. Lim AKP et al. Embolization of bleeding residual uterine vascular malformations in patients with treated gestational trophoblastic tumors. Radiology. 2002;222:640–4.
46. Mangili G et al. Trophoblastic disease review for diagnosis and management: A joint report from the international society for the study of trophoblastic disease, European organisation for the treatment of trophoblastic disease, and the gynecologic cancer InterGroup. Int J Gynecol Cancer. 2014;24:S109–16.
47. Tonorezos E et al. Prevalence of cancer survivors in the United States. J Natl Cancer Inst. 2024;116(11):1784–90.
48. Cronin KA et al. Annual report to the nation on the status of cancer, part 1: National cancer statistics. Cancer. 2022;128(24):4251–84.
49. Peerenboom R et al. Surviving and thriving: What do survivors of gynecologic cancer want? Gynecol Oncol Rep. 2022;41:101011.
50. Woopen H et al. GCIG-consensus guideline for long-term survivorship in gynecologic cancer: A position paper from the gynecologic cancer Intergroup (GCIG) symptom benefit committee. Cancer Treat Rev. 2022;107:102396.
51. Lokich E. Gynecologic cancer survivorship. Obstet Gynecol Clin North Am. 2019;46:165–78.
52. Boakye EA et al. Risk of second primary cancers among survivors of gynecological cancers. Gynecol Oncol. 2020;158(3):719–26.

53. Campbell KM, Rodríguez JE. Addressing the minority tax: Perspectives from two diversity leaders on building minority faculty success in academic medicine. Acad Med. 2019;94:1854–57.

54. Rock CL et al. Nutrition and physical activity guidelines for cancer survivors. CA Cancer J Clin. 2012;62(4):243–74.

55. Agnew H et al. Interventions for weight reduction in obesity to improve survival in women with endometrial cancer. Cochrane Database Syst Rev. 2023;CD012513.pub3.

56. McCarroll ML et al. Self-efficacy, quality of life, and weight loss in overweight/obese endometrial cancer survivors (SUCCEED): A randomized controlled trial. Gynecol Oncol. 2014;132(2):397–402.

57. Smits A et al. The effect of lifestyle interventions on the quality of life of gynaecological cancer survivors: A systematic review and meta-analysis. Gynecol Oncol. 2015;139(3):546–52.

58. Wang L et al. Glucagon-like peptide 1 receptor agonists and 13 obesity-associated cancers in patients with type 2 diabetes. JAMA Netw Open. 2024;7(7):e2421305.

59. Pati S et al. Obesity and cancer: A current overview of epidemiology, pathogenesis, outcomes, and management. Cancers. 2023;15(2):485.

60. Robertson MC et al. Change in physical activity and quality of life in endometrial cancer survivors receiving a physical activity intervention. Health Qual Life Outcomes. 2019;17(1):91.

61. Koutoukidis DA et al. Diet, physical activity, and health-related outcomes of endometrial cancer survivors in a behavioral lifestyle program: The diet and exercise in uterine cancer survivors (DEUS) parallel randomized controlled pilot trial. Int J Gynecol Cancer. 2019;29(3):531–40.

62. Viamonte SG et al. Cardio-oncology rehabilitation for cancer survivors with high cardiovascular risk: A randomized clinical trial. JAMA Cardiol. 2023;1;8(12):1119–28.

63. Xu J et al. A systematic review of dietary interventions for cancer survivors and their families or caregivers. Nutrients. 2023 Dec 23;16(1):56.

64. Bower JE. Cancer-related fatigue—mechanisms, risk factors, and treatments. Nat Rev Clin Oncol. 2014;11:597–609.

65. Westin SN et al. Survivors of gynecologic malignancies: Impact of treatment on health and well-being. J Cancer Surviv. 2016;10(2):261–70.

66. Sekse RJ et al. Fatigue and quality of life in women treated for various types of gynaecological cancers: A cross-sectional study. J Clin Nurs. 2015;24(3–4):546–55.

67. Poort H et al. Patterns and predictors of cancer-related fatigue in ovarian and endometrial cancers: 1-year longitudinal study. Cancer. 2020;1;126(15):3526–33.

68. Bower JE et al. Management of fatigue in adult survivors of cancer: ASCO-society for integrative oncology guideline update. J Clin Oncol. 2024;10;42(20):2456–87.

69. Yu CH et al. Healthy life styles, sleep and fatigue in endometrial cancer survivors: A cross-sectional study. J Clin Nurs. 2020;29(7–8):1372–80.

70. Bennett S et al. Educational interventions for the management of cancer-related fatigue in adults. Cochrane Database Syst Rev. 2016;CD008144.pub2.

71. Lin H et al. Evaluation of sexual dysfunction in gynecologic cancer survivors using DSM-5 diagnostic criteria. BMC Womens Health. 2022;22(1):1.

72. Abbott-Anderson K, Kwekkeboom KL. A systematic review of sexual concerns reported by gynecological cancer survivors. Gynecol Oncol. 2012;124:477–89.

73. Chang CP et al. Sexual dysfunction among gynecologic cancer survivors in a population-based cohort study. Support Care Cancer. 2022;17;31(1):51.

74. Goetsch MF et al. A practical solution for dyspareunia in breast cancer survivors: A randomized controlled trial. J Clin Oncol. 2015;33:3394–400.

75. Hinds L, Price J. Menopause, hormone replacement and gynaecological cancers. Menopause Int. 2010;16(2):89–93.

76. Pergialiotis V et al. Hormone therapy for ovarian cancer survivors: Systematic review and meta-analysis. Menopause. 2016;23:335–42.

77. Barakat RR et al. Randomized double-blind trial of estrogen replacement therapy versus placebo in stage I or II endometrial cancer: A gynecologic oncology group study. J Clin Oncol. 2006;24:587–92.

78. Ploch E. Hormonal replacement therapy in patients after cervical cancer treatment. Gynecol Oncol. 1987;26:169–77.

79. Vargiu V et al. Hormone replacement therapy and cervical cancer: A systematic review of the literature. Climacteric. 2021;24:120–7.
80. Rauh LA et al. Hormone replacement therapy after treatment for cervical cancer: Are we adhering to standard of care? Gynecol Oncol. 2017;147:597–600.
81. Haest K et al. Stellate ganglion block for the management of hot flashes and sleep disturbances in breast cancer survivors: An uncontrolled experimental study with 24 weeks of follow-up. Ann Oncol. 2012;23(6):1449–54.
82. Deng G et al. Randomized, controlled trial of acupuncture for the treatment of hot flashes in breast cancer patients. J Clin Oncol. 2007;10;25(35):5584–90.
83. Maclaughlan DS et al. Randomised controlled trial comparing hypnotherapy versus gabapentin for the treatment of hot flashes in breast cancer survivors: A pilot study. BMJ Open. 2013;3:e003138.
84. Campbell G et al. Caring for survivors of gynecologic cancer: Assessment and management of long-term and late effects. Semin Oncol Nurs. 2019;35(2):192–201. doi:10.1016/j.soncn.2019.02.006.
85. Ramaseshan AS et al. Pelvic floor disorders in women with gynecologic malignancies: A systematic review. Int Urogynecol J. 2018;29(4):459–76.
86. Seretny M et al. Incidence, prevalence, and predictors of chemotherapy-induced peripheral neuropathy: A systematic review and meta-analysis. Pain. 2014;155(12):2461–70.
87. Loprinzi CL et al. Prevention and management of chemotherapy-induced peripheral neuropathy in survivors of adult cancers: ASCO guideline update. J Clin Oncol. 2020;1;38(28):3325–48.
88. Cao A et al. Effect of exercise on chemotherapy-induced peripheral neuropathy among patients treated for ovarian cancer: A secondary analysis of a randomized clinical trial. JAMA Netw Open. 2023;1;6(8):e2326463.
89. Hartung TJ et al. The risk of being depressed is significantly higher in cancer patients than in the general population: Prevalence and severity of depressive symptoms across major cancer types. Eur J Cancer. 2017;72:46–53.
90. Watts S et al. Depression and anxiety in ovarian cancer: A systematic review and meta-analysis of prevalence rates. BMJ Open. 2015 Nov 30;5(11):e007618.
91. Andersen BL et al. Management of anxiety and depression in adult survivors of cancer: ASCO guideline update. J Clin Oncol. 2023;41(18):3426–53.
92. Simard S et al. Fear of cancer recurrence in adult cancer survivors: A systematic review of quantitative studies. J Cancer Surviv. 2013;7:300–22.
93. Luigjes-Huizer YL et al. What is the prevalence of fear of cancer recurrence in cancer survivors and patients? A systematic review and individual participant data meta-analysis. Psychooncology. 2022;31(6):879–92.
94. Mell CA et al. Psychosocial predictors of fear of cancer recurrence in a cohort of gynecologic cancer survivors. Psychooncology. 2022;31(12):2141–8.
95. Götze H et al. Fear of cancer recurrence across the survivorship trajectory: Results from a survey of adult long-term cancer survivors. Psychooncology. 2019;28(10):2033–41.
96. Tauber NM et al. Effect of psychological intervention on fear of cancer recurrence: A systematic review and meta-analysis. J Clin Oncol. 2019;37(31):2899–915.

Index

Note: Page numbers in *italics* indicate a figure and page numbers in **bold** indicate a table on the corresponding page.

For Product Safety Concerns and Information please contact our EU
representative GPSR@taylorandfrancis.com
Taylor & Francis Verlag GmbH, Kaufingerstraße 24, 80331 München, Germany

www.ingramcontent.com/pod-product-compliance
Lightning Source LLC
Chambersburg PA
CBHW081537220326
41598CB00036B/6468